I CO[illegible] FIBROMYALGIA

AND TURNED

HORROR MOANS

BACK INTO

HORMONES

Pam Fitzgerald and Linda Yates

Disclaimer:

Pam Fitzgerald and Linda Yates are not medical doctors. This is Pam's story on how she conquered Fibromyalgia. Please consult your physician before any treatment.

www.iconqueredfibromyalgia.com

ISBN 0-9703916-0-9

First Printing - August, 2000

Printed by

Laborde Printing Company, Inc.
New Orleans, Louisiana

DEDICATION

I wholeheartedly dedicate this book to my family—for support and unconditional love—my beloved husband, John, my loving children, Candace and Seth, and my wonderful son-in-law, Edward.

They were by my side through my pain and suffering.

They often suffered along with me by giving up their own activities to assist me. I am forever grateful and thank God everyday that he gave us all the precious gift of life and that he blessed my life with such a wonderful family.

They were always there for me and never treated me like a burden; this somehow gave me the courage and determination to find a way out of this imprisonment of pain.

I love them all!

And Daddy was not here in person, but he was in my heart and thoughts encouraging me to go on. I miss him.

CONTENTS

PREFACE

Fibromyalgia Syndrome—there are various theories as to its cause. None have been proven. There are corresponding attempts at treatment. My explanation of the syndrome is hormone imbalance. Further, I have found that the bioidentical hormones, not the synthetic ones, are effective in controlling my condition. The indication is that this may be true for other sufferers as well. I hope that this book offers new possibilities to some readers for the improvement of their own conditions.

Although I have learned ways to control my fibromyalgia, as well as other symptoms of hormonal imbalance, I did not accomplish this without help and guidance. There are several physicians who have been instrumental in my success. Without their compassion, their acceptance of me and my puzzling symptoms, their encouragement and prodding, their patience to listen to all I had to say, and especially their support of my suggestions for alternative treatments, I would have given up. They are truly wonderful individuals. This book is a testament to the effectiveness of their efforts. They will recognize that this is true because, repeatedly, they saw my hopelessness.

My heartfelt thanks go out to Dr. Thomas Givens, Dr. Richard Strub, Dr. Robert Quinet, Dr. John Milek, Dr. Demarcus Smith, and Dr. Michael Flynn. They are certainly above average in their profession. Not only through healing arts, but also through human kindness, they are truly serving the needs of their patients.

ACKNOWLEDGMENTS

First of all, I would like to say that my co-author has truly been a very important asset in the writing of this book. She was a very knowledgeable schoolteacher and has kept me on track, correcting my wording and punctuation—sometimes as though I were still in school. She helped me to refine my words and she studied and learned a lot about fibromyalgia in a short period of time. Thanks, Linda, for believing in me enough to devote over a year of your life to this project. And thanks to her husband Bill, her daughter Kim, her family, and Bobbie Barker for their support and help.

Next, I would like to take the opportunity to thank the one who made my life possible in the first place. Mom, you were there through all the ups and downs, and you are a true example of what a mom should be. Thanks for the many meals and love and support through this project.

Candy and Edward, my daughter and son-in-law, helped with the picture sections as model and photographer. Edward also rescued us from our many computer glitches. I am very grateful and feel indebted to them both.

The book would have been finished much later if not for the loving help of my siblings. I had lots of help thanks to Mom and Dad who provided eight of them—I agree with that old saying, "Eight is enough." But I thank my sisters and brothers, especially the scrabble players, from the bottom of my heart for their loyal support.

I could call on my best friend Mona day or night. She has always been there whenever or for whatever I needed her. Thank you, Butterfly.

And my husband's uncle, who lives with us, is my "adopted" son. I tease him a lot. Thank you, Cliff, for helping with the chores and cooking; the help was greatly appreciated.

I want to thank a very special lady, Mrs. Darby, who came into my life when I needed help and encouragement. She became a second mother to me and really needs to be thanked from the bottom of my heart.

And last, but not least, I want to thank a very loyal and excellent employee at our local Office Max. Archie, I really appreciate you helping me get out manuscripts to the many places we needed to. You were always willing to go out of your way to finish whatever we needed even if we were last minute walk-ins. You are a valuable asset to your company and the customers there.

Author's Notes

It is amazing how complex a creation the human body is. In this book I do not go into specific scientific detail about chemical processes. But I do want to just mention a few of the processes in our bodies that I think affect fibromyalgia.

Our cells make up all of the tissues of the body. Cells carry out all of the body's functional activities, and cell structure and form is closely correlated with the job of the cell.

Enzymes are proteins that serve as catalysts for chemical reactions in cells; these chemical reactions are a part of metabolism or metabolic processes. Metabolism is the sum of all physical and chemical changes that take place within the body. The body's ability for correct metabolism affects all bodily functions, including the production and use of hormones. Hormones are chemical messengers that stimulate organs to increase or to decrease activity or to increase or decrease secretion of other hormones.

Neurotransmitters are also very important to the body and to fibromyalgia patients. They relay messages from one neuron (brain cell) to another. I agree with the theory that in FMS the neurotransmitters are disrupted and this causes other disturbances in the body. Our HPA axis—hypothalamus, pituitary and adrenal glands--communicate by way of neurotransmitters. The loss of estrogen is one cause of disruption in the HPA axis. Neurotransmitters are affected by the chemical reactions of enzymes and hormones.

The bottom line is that the chemicals that get into and onto your body in the form of medicine or food or environmental elements can have very big effects (good and bad) on the body. If your body is "out of whack" then look at these things for the source.

INTRODUCTION

These are probably the most sincere and heartfelt writings and feelings that any person has ever written. My mind is so invigorated and my heart is so at peace. I only wish that twenty years ago someone with experiences like mine had shared them in writing as I am doing now for you.

I am not a doctor or a trained professional, but **I am a survivor with considerably less pain.** I am educated in Fibromyalgia Syndrome (FMS) and in pain, especially as these pertain to me. Had I studied this long and hard in a university, I could probably have a degree by now. Some people say that they majored in math or in history. I can say I majored in fibromyalgia and pain, and I have learned to control FMS much more than it controls me.

Fibromyalgia Syndrome is a painful, confusing and frustrating condition. It has taken over my thought processes, my goals, my time, and my money for most of my adult life. It caused me to feel like a prisoner locked up in my own body. I was screaming to be released so that I could be a wife, mother, and friend to the many people that I loved and wanted to be with, but nobody was hearing me.

My symptoms were life changing. I wandered from doctor to doctor for years aimlessly looking for relief. I endured many unnecessary and very hurtful medications, medical tests, treatments, and surgeries, and I am still paying the physical price for some of them. There was little knowledge in the medical field to help me. Doctors, friends, and sometimes even my family thought I was fabricating excuses—in medical books it is called malingering. Doctors frequently told me that nothing was wrong, that it was all in my head. (Many fibromites will acknowledge that they had to visit many doctors before finding one who did not treat them as if they were mentally unbalanced.) After years of misdiagnosis, no diagnosis, and treatments which either had no effect or which made my condition worse, I had just about given up on having any kind of life. I finally felt so hopeless that I started seriously studying the procedures for disability status. I even discussed it with my doctor.

One day, at Ochsner Clinic in New Orleans, I was finally given a name for the years of pain and other chronic symptoms. That day marked the beginning of my personal attempt to study and to conquer FMS. Having a name gave me the ability to focus my search for a cure. I did not realize what an extensive search it would become. I became motivated to take control and to learn all that I could about my condition. I began to study for myself and not just depend on doctors.

I have now spent years studying. I have talked with (and paid) countless doctors. I have searched actively. I have read books, articles, and anything else I could find. This has been a very difficult education. Although I feel that I now have some understanding of *my* fibromyalgia, the literature I've seen says that the medical and scientific communities still do not understand it very well. More studies are under way now, so progress is being made and there is reason for hope.

Not only did I study the literature, I studied my body. I studied my reactions to everything, physical and emotional. I was persistent and determined. I noted times, types, and triggers of pain. I studied the pharmaceutical literature given to me with my prescription medications and asked pharmacists for more. I worked with the amount and timing of drug doses. I tried conventional and alternative therapies.

However, getting to the point of writing a book, instead of accepting permanent disability, is the result of a series of coincidences. These coincidental events proved my original belief that hormone imbalance had some role in my FMS. That led to the connection of bioidentical hormones to my disease. My positive bodily reaction to bioidentical hormones has been the most important key and the biggest surprise. I actually am having good days after many years of daily awakening to pain and closing my eyes to pain. I am continually getting even better, instead of having my health deteriorate, because I am better attuned to my body. I have been able to resume many activities that I thought were lost to me forever. I want to make clear just how much better my life is now, even though for years the pain of FMS had been constant and severe. I have learned how to control, and even usually avoid, flare-ups. So, although I still have it, I feel so much better that I almost want to deny ever having been diagnosed with fibromyalgia.

My very difficult journey for the past years in this health battle titled "fibromyalgia" has taken a complete turn around. I am very elated with my new health status, and that is the main reason for writing this book. I want to share my success. My goal is to help prevent the bad things that happened to me from happening to anyone else. Through many years of pain and perseverance, I have found such an abundance of relief that I am bubbling over to share with anyone suffering from this life-altering malady. I want to share hard-won knowledge with the hope that you might also enjoy a dramatic change in your pain cycle, and that this change might give you your old self back as it has done for me. I want to tell you how I got to this point. My wish is that you become assured that you can control the pain of fibromyalgia.

While reading this book, remember that it represents my own very personal experiences. It is written from my own point of view. It is not meant to be a complete study of Fibromyalgia Syndrome. That is a job for professionals. Research on fibromyalgia is barely getting started and there is new information all the time. Some of it is beginning to support my theory, but there are several other theories as well.

Included in the chapters are detailed explanations that could possibly help a person desperate for pain relief. I have explained how I came to know or to believe certain things about the syndrome. I have described methods and tactics for experimenting with ideas, therapies and medications. Many of the methods are ones I developed by trial and error after miserable results from other ones prescribed for me. By describing these trial and error processes, I hope to help you control your pain in a shorter time than I did. You may want to try some of the things included in this book, and I think many of them will work for you. But in addition to trying my methods, a major goal here is to show you how experimentation led to better results for me. I hope that as you read what did, or did not, work for me, you will be encouraged to experiment (with the help of your doctor) with your own therapies and medications, while staying safe and more comfortable in the process.

The books that I have mentioned helped me immensely, and I think they will help you, too. Doctors and patients have written many of the books, and these are the ones to take to your doctor if you wish to suggest a treatment not previously considered. Moreover, my information is not just from books, but also from booklets or pamphlets from medical institutions and associations, as well as from TV shows, news articles, and other sources.

Reading my story should demonstrate just how important good doctors are to the successful management of fibromyalgia. It made all the difference to me when I found doctors who would work *with* me instead of *on* me. It helped, too, when I learned to think of myself as the captain of the team and to think of the doctor, the pharmacist, and my family as team members. More doctors are beginning to accept this approach and some of them even invite input about treatments from their patients. Less often do they discredit or condemn patients who report to them the use of alternative therapies or supplements. Increasingly, doctors are using alternative treatments themselves.

And, concerning doctors, all of that studying I did has substantially paid off. I can now go to a doctor and hear "You may be right," or "You're absolutely right." However, it still takes an open-minded doctor (I found some out there) to say such things. If I have a suggestion for my own treatment, doctors are more likely to listen, to guide me, and to help me monitor the effects. One doctor told me he had never seen an FMS patient with such positive results as mine. I have even had doctors in separate specialties ask me if they might have a friend or a patient with fibromyalgia call me for advice on pain management.

So please, if you are suffering the awful symptoms of fibromyalgia, don't give up, but follow me through my experiences and see what wonderful changes can lie ahead for you. My heart wants to help each and every one of you because I have been there and I know what it is like to feel lost in the many, many files of many, many doctors with treatments that lead you nowhere near any sign of relief. I know what it is like to try each new thing thinking that you have the answer, and then to backslide in the realization that you had false hopes. There is an answer for each of you, and I feel that if you try some of the things I suggest, you will be amazed at how much you will be able to put the syndrome out of your mind longer and longer each day.

CHAPTER ONE

FIBROMYALGIA SYNDROME

FMS

DEFINITION AND STATISTICS

What is fibromyalgia? The struggle to deal with it has disrupted my life for over a decade. I think that anyone with this condition would agree that this is the sixty-four-thousand dollar question. Dr. Charles Mary, M.D., former head of Charity Hospital in New Orleans, defined it in a recent WTIX radio talk show (9-1-99). He described fibro (connective tissue) my (muscle) algia (ache) as a condition similar to rheumatoid arthritis. It is a disease that involves various kinds of chronic pains or aches throughout the body. Medical tests cannot detect or explain it. Usually, there are other ailments present at the same time. It is considered a disease of the arthritis family of disorders, and the Arthritis Foundation has formulated information for the public in *Your Personal Guide to Living Well with Fibromyalgia (1997)*.

"Syndrome" is the term given to this condition because a group of different symptoms, not just one simple symptom, is involved in fibromyalgia, and because there is no known single cause or etiology. Syndrome is defined in *Taber's Cyclopedic Medical Dictionary* (1997):

> A group of symptoms and signs of disordered function related to one another by means of some anatomical, physiological, or biochemical peculiarity. This definition does not include a precise cause of an illness but does provide a framework of reference for investigating it.

In fact, there are several theories being tested about the cause of FMS, but none have been conclusive. For now, we must be content with symptom abatement without complete understanding.

A growing number of people are given the diagnosis of Fibromyalgia Syndrome every day. In *Parade* (7-18-99), Dr. Isadore Rosenfeld has said that six million Americans are afflicted. How many more people might not yet be diagnosed? Estimates vary, but some say that women account for as many as ninety percent of the cases. Victims are usually between twenty and forty years old.

HISTORY

Although fibromyalgia syndrome appears to be a quite new phenomenon in medical practice, Miryam Williamson in *Fibromyalgia: A Comprehensive Approach*, describes a possible long history for this disease. She says that physicians have recorded a condition involving many FMS symptoms since the early 1800s; they called it muscular rheumatism. In 1824, an Edinburgh doctor described tender points. Williamson says that in 1880 an American psychiatrist blamed modern lifestyle stresses for a condition he called neurasthenia that involved general fatigue, widespread pain, and psychological disturbance. Perhaps that is the reason so many women were sent to insane asylums in those early days.

Fibromyalgia seems to be more common now—6,000,000 Americans with the diagnosis. Because the symptoms are varied and confusing, it has been misdiagnosed for a long time. In fact, it has been ignored in the medical community for years. Doctors have tended, and still often do so, to attribute the symptoms to mental problems, especially in women. There is progress. The Rosenfeld article (*Parade, 7-18-99)* states that the international medical community accepted FMS as a real disease entity in 1993. Also, Devin Starlanyl, M.D., and Mary Ellen Copeland, MS, MA, (*Fibromyalgia & Chronic Myofascial Pain Syndrome: A Survival Manual)* say that the American Medical Association (AMA) officially recognized the disease in 1987.

Fibromyalgia has been known by various names over the decades. An older common name was fibrocitis, which was changed when it became apparent that inflammation (itis) is not a factor. Fibromyositis was also used some. Any name for the condition, however, was progress. A copy of the 10th edition (1965) of *Tabor's Cyclopedic Medical Dictionary* does not even list fibrositis. (Notice how closely this date coincides with the wide release of birth control hormone pills--no fibrocitis in the books before 1965.)

Some medical dictionaries and medical encyclopedias still, in 1999, do not have fibromyalgia listed in their pages. Many still list only the term fibrositis. The new 1999 Merck Manual discusses "Primary Fibromyalgia Syndrome" (PFS). And some of the newest dictionaries and encyclopedias discuss FMS in the plural--syndromes. The terminology seems to be changing and narrowing as the understanding changes. I did my own casual search for these terms in the newest books at several of the local bookstores, and I can tell you that "official" information is still scarce and sometimes lagging even today.

TERMINOLOGY AND LINGO

When the name, fibromyalgia, is mentioned, most people still get a quizzical look on their faces and admit to total ignorance of the term. However, it is becoming recognized more often now. People are beginning to know the word because they know someone with FMS. There are even some special terms and lingo developing concerning FMS.

In *Fibromyalgia and Chronic Myofascial Pain Syndrome: A Survival Manual* (Starlanyl and Copeland, 1996) I found the coined terms "fibromite" and "fibrofog." Fibromite is the term for a victim of fibromyalgia. She or he has been to scores of doctors and has spent thousands of dollars looking for relief—at least that is the tale of every fibromite I know or have read about. Fibrofog denotes the fuzzy, confused feeling that can afflict fibromites, especially when they wake up in the morning. Fibrofog can be short term or it can last for months; I related to this term immediately. A "flare" or flare-up can occur at any time. These authors point out that all symptoms are amplified during a flare-up. New and old symptoms may appear together, and the episode is "all-consuming." I agree.

Tender points and trigger points are often confused. They are confused both linguistically and diagnostically. You will see the term used differently in different medical books, and not all doctors distinguish them correctly in their language or in their diagnoses. I have taken my descriptions from many sources, including personal experiences; I've included a chart. The Starlanyl/Copeland book is very descriptive as well.

Tender points are fixed points on the body that are designated by medical authorities as indicators of fibromyalgia. There are eighteen of these tender points, and they are in symmetrical pairs, at points from the neck to the knees. You might respond to pain when, and only when, any one of the points is pressed. Some are on the front and some are on the back of the body. It hurts when a tender point is pressed, but pain is not referred or sent to other areas of the body. A fibromite may not be aware of a tender point until it is pressed, but most authorities agree that the point will hurt every time it is pressed during the course of the illness.

Trigger points (TrPs) are indicative of myofascial pain syndrome (MPS), and not of FMS, according to Starlanyl and Copeland (1996). MPS is a disorder of the fascia (lining) of the muscles. More often than not, FMS and MPS are experienced together, so the symptoms can overlap. Unlike tender points, a person might have trigger points almost anywhere in the body, including near or with tender points. That can make it very hard for even the most experienced doctor to distinguish them. But, a person can have many, many trigger points, not just eighteen. They can be present in just one place, or in several areas. Trigger points are notorious for referring pain to other, sometimes seemingly separate, parts of the body. With correct therapies, trigger points can be eliminated, which is not the case with tender points.

SYMPTOMS AND ASSOCIATED AILMENTS

You will be interested to see what symptoms other fibromites have experienced if you are diagnosed with fibromyalgia. Knowing what might be expected can serve as a guide when you talk to your doctor. It can also lend a measure of mental comfort.

What are the symptoms that might cause you to consider fibromyalgia as a possible cause for pains and other problems you are having? Of course, it is impossible to diagnose yourself. You absolutely must have a doctor to help you pin down the cause of your problems because there are so many maladies which cause the same, or similar, symptoms. Some of these "other maladies" are easy to control or cure. You surely do not want to "give yourself" a worse disease than you really have--and sometimes human nature causes us to fear the worst. That could cause you many additional problems. On the other hand, and just as important, neither do you want to think that you have something simple, or nothing at all, when you really have a serious condition that needs treatment. An accurate diagnosis is very, very important.

The most notable symptom is body pain, specific sometimes, but more often unspecified. If body aches that won't quit are not enough, there is quite a list of ailments that may be present along with FMS. Myofascial Pain Syndrome is one; in fact, it is listed in the FMS entries in some of the later medical literature. Chronic Fatigue Syndrome, and Irritable Bowel Syndrome are also notorious cohorts that frequently show up with FMS. Many patients have digestive problems. Food sensitivity and allergies are common. Most suffer sleep disturbances and chronic fatigue. Hypothyroidism and mitral valve prolapse can be troublesome. I had them all and continuously tried to find some sort of relief. With so many abstract and "incurable" symptoms to cope with and for such long periods, it is little wonder that one woman turned to Dr. Kavorkian because she felt she had no way out. However, only in very bad instances will all of the symptoms show up at the same time; although, in a flare-up it is not unusual to have many of them at the same time.

FMS has treated me badly. I had widespread pain throughout my muscles; my joints ached; and I had severe lower back pain, pelvic pain, leg cramps, and stiffness in the neck and shoulders. The pain in my legs I can only describe as feeling like severe toothaches; there was a burning pain, and I felt like my legs were going to explode. Migraines tormented me two or three times a week. I had stomach problems, indigestion, diarrhea, and nausea. I experienced heart palpitations that were later diagnosed as mitral valve prolapse. This condition involves a bulging heart valve that allows the blood to flow backwards during a heartbeat. It is a problem common to FMS patients.

Fatigue plagued me, and sleep disturbances were a daily part of my life, as is often the case for fibromites. I felt extreme fatigue no matter what supplements I used, including B-12 injections. I could not get comfortable enough to fall asleep, so I would stay awake until two or three o'clock in the morning. When I did fall asleep, I would wake up easily and often. On these occasions, I would resist getting up or moving too much for fear of initiating pain. In the mornings I would wake up and not want to move an inch because the moment I moved, the pain would begin. From being in constant pain, I felt like I had a dark cloud hanging over me all the time. My mornings were a confused slow-motion affair. This was fibrofog.

Have you ever been told that you have fibrofog? It felt as though I had not slept for a week. I felt so tired and sleepy. I was so weak that I found it hard to get up. I would try so hard to wake up, then get up, and then accomplish what I had planned for the day. I could hardly think, much less focus and concentrate on demanding tasks.

Awakening to pain, my days would begin with pain in my neck, shoulders, jaw, and legs. I would walk stiffly to the bathroom and try so hard to get ready for work. The first thing I would have to do was to take half of a pain pill and a Zantac to protect my stomach because it was always so irritated from all of the anti-inflammatory drugs I had taken. I tried ice packs, heating pads, and hot showers. They helped the stiffness, but they did not shake the horrible feelings of fibrofog in the mornings.

It became a joke that I was not a morning person, but I just felt so fatigued every morning. I began my quest to find energy in a bottle. I tried all kinds of vitamin supplements and medications. No matter what I tried I was always tired. I did not find much relief until I began using the magnets and bioidentical hormones.

DIAGNOSIS

Many and quite varied diagnoses have been given to explain my pain, headaches, and other problems. To obtain these many diagnoses, I have undergone unnecessary tests and surgeries--some tests were just as painful as the surgeries. I wish there were some way to go back and just start over.

At first everything was blamed on STRESS! That opinion was so prevalent that some of my family, friends, co-workers, and even the doctors acted as if they thought my pain was all in my head. Stress is a factor, but it is not the only factor, and the pain of FMS is very real. Some doctors ignored or denied the existence of the pain. Believe it or not, there are still some doctors who think it is just all in a patient's mind. I had a fellow FMS patient tell me that a doctor made that very statement to her just recently. Where has he been? Evidently, he must not know anyone with this very painful condition! Or, for that matter, he must not be keeping up with the latest medical studies.

Perhaps, the medical profession first blamed stress because stress can cause flare-ups. But I resented the fact that most doctors only wanted to put me on nerve pills for stress, and they neglected to even consider the reason for the pain. I strongly resisted using the nerve pills. I am now approaching my forty-fourth birthday and I can honestly say that I now know what stress is. It is being told that you have fibromyalgia and then beginning treatment after treatment after treatment for it and searching and searching for any kind of relief.

Part of the diagnosis of fibromyalgia, early on and now, involves ruling out other diseases with similar symptoms. Lupus, Lyme Disease, hypoglycemia and hypothyroidism are examples. There is no blood test to detect fibromyalgia. When tests are given, they usually read normal.

The only real way to diagnose FMS is from the symptoms (see chart at the end of this section). The accepted test is to locate tender points on the body. There are eighteen precise tender points that doctors look for and I reacted to all eighteen. If a person responds to eleven (sometimes fewer) of the eighteen tender points, if the pain response to the tender points falls in all four quadrants of the body, if the pain has persisted for at least three months, and if there are other designated symptoms, then the diagnosis of fibromyalgia is given.

What about my own diagnosis? About ten years ago, at Ochsner Clinic in New Orleans, I was finally diagnosed with a disease with a name instead of someone just trying to blame this on STRESS. (I have come to hate that word.) I had Fibrositis! As the doctor told me what I had, I began to sob, so relieved that someone was finally going to help me. By that time I had spent thousands and thousands of dollars and endured painful tests, treatments, and surgeries--all to no avail. But I finally had a specific name for my symptoms. I thought that meant that there was a specific treatment, with specific results. Little did I know that FMS was so complicated, and so misunderstood in the medical profession, that it really had the doctors as confused as the patients.

Tender Points:

There are eighteen spicific tenderpoints on the body:

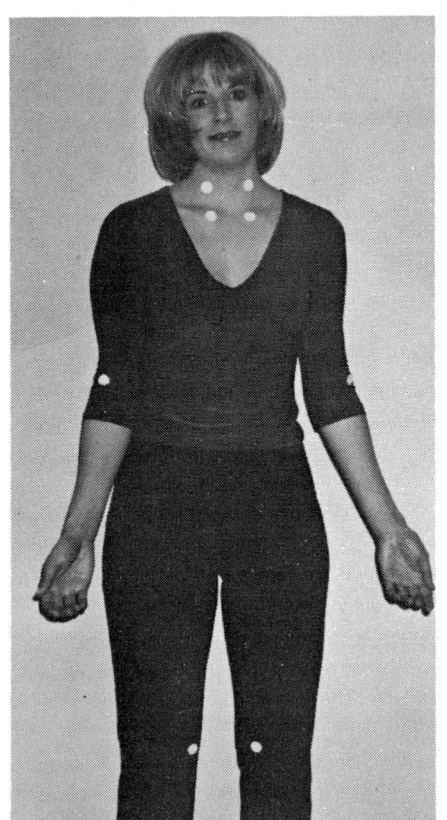

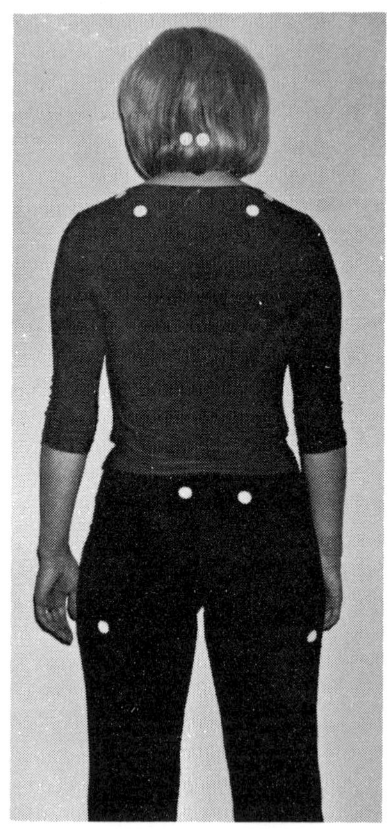

A usual diagnosis is at least eleven tender points present in the four quadrants of the body for an accurate diagnosis!

CAUSES AND CURE

The cause of fibromyalgia remains a mystery, although new theories are being studied. There is no known cure. However, I believe that my experience directs the way to such complete control that I can at least call it remission if not a cure.

What causes FMS and why has this "new" ailment surfaced now? Fibromyalgia does seem more widespread in recent years. That may be partly because medical diagnosis is so much more advanced now.. That is, fibromyalgia stands out as a separate disease now, whereas in the past it did not. As Williamson suggested, it has been around, just missed.

The 1999 Merck Manual states no known cause for FMS, but says that it can be "exacerbated" by physical or emotional stress. It lists the usual other syndromes as factors. It also lists, and I quote, "uncaring doctors who give the patient the message that it is 'all in the head'."

A possible causative factor I wish to offer is the birth control pill and HRT using synthetic hormones. Rresearch may later show that the pill caused many cases of FMS; those early birth control preparations were much, much stronger than the ones given today. Also, hormone replacement therapy has changed a lot since its beginning. It is becoming obvious that the medical community over prescribes synthetic hormones—doctors give hormones to women who do not need them, and they give doses that are too strong or too large to many women who may need them. The medical community is in fact reevaluating the dosages of hormones commonly given to women. In a recent radio program (WTIX in New Orleans), Dr. Charles Mary, who favors bioidentical hormones, told one caller that women who take synthetic estrogen seem to have higher than normal incidences of FMS. An experience I had points to his conclusion. One lady heard about me and called; she had symptoms of FMS. I suggested that she ask her doctor about the possibility of fibromyalgia; he did diagnose FMS. With the help of her doctor, she stopped using Premarin, used some of my victory plan, started taking nutritional supplements, and she now reports that she is doing much better and has her life back.

Other factors may include environmental issues. Researchers at Tulane University Medical Center and Ochsner Medical Foundation are conducting a study to determine whether environmental factors may cause fibromyalgia. Increasingly, contaminated environment is being blamed for hormone imbalance and there are indications that we have more hormone imbalance problems than our ancestors did. Dr. John R. Lee, Dr. Jesse Hanley, and Virginia Hopkins tell us in *What Your Doctor May Not Tell You about Premenopause* (1999) that estrogens and xenohormones are present in our daily lives in countless hidden ways. These agents act like estrogen in the human body and are unbalancing hormones in the whole population (pp. 41, 51). They are in the meats; they are in soaps, carpets, building materials, plastics, pesticides, and on and on (p.48); they are even in milk. Dr. Lee and his co-authors attribute many of today's ills to these environmental xenohormones; they call the phenomenon estrogen dominance. Estrogen dominance, they say, is rampant in our modern existence. They cause infertility, arthritis, and untold other chronic problems. I would add fibromyalgia to the list based on the hindsight view of my experiences with pain and hormones.

Such ideas are popping up in other places, too. Medical programs and news media are increasingly airing spots on the subject of environmental issues and hormones. This demonstrates public suspicions that hormone imbalance may be an important factor in many health problems. Examples of this creeping awareness can be seen in the increasing numbers of advertisements for soy and other herbal products (with phytohormones) for menopausal women; these have increased noticeably even in the last six months.

The causes of my own fibromyalgia? I may never be completely sure, but as I look back over my medical history, I see what seem to be significant factors that point to hormone imbalance. I began having problems as soon as I began menstruating. A car accident when I was twenty started my body pains. In fact, I believe that the wreck may have contributed to my fibromyalgia along with my already existing hormone and sleeping disorder. During my two pregnancies, I felt wonderful. After the pregnancies, the symptoms returned, especially after the second birth when I began to take birth control pills. This makes me believe that my hormones were more balanced during these pregnancies and that is why my suffering disappeared then.

CONVENTIONAL TREATMENTS

There is so much controversy over the treatment of fibromyalgia, and with good reason. How can a doctor treat something that nobody yet understands. It is little wonder that we have been misdiagnosed, mistreated, and ignored in the medical field. In fact, some of my treatments and surgeries caused very serious problems leading to more treatments and surgeries. Some of these have left me with bad symptoms that will affect me the rest of my life. It is my opinion that several of my treatments and surgeries could have been avoided, had understanding of the disorder, and of hormones, been clear. But, the medical community has just begun to be confronted with the syndrome, and many doctors just do not know anything about it. My TMJ surgery is an example—after three and a half years of prescriptions and the subsequent TMJ surgery, that same doctor, who was an extremely caring person, referred me to the doctor who diagnosed fibrocitis. Again, I'll refer to Dr. Charles Mary who recently told a caller to the radio show (WTIX, New Orleans, La.) that some FMS treatments can be dangerous.

The most common prescription for fibromyalgia is anti-inflammatory medication. This is usually accompanied by an anti-depressant, often Elavil. Some doctors prescribe pain medications and muscle relaxing agents as well. Most of the medications have possible side effects that can be serious. Some of the drugs I have been prescribed over these years are: Valium, Flexeril, Librax, Pamelor, Inderal, Tenorman, Elavil, Relefen, Soma, Ultram, Zoloft, Xanax, Midrin, Imitrex, Diflucan, Zomig, Colestid, Zantac, Pepcid, Desyrel, Celebrix, Naprosyn, Lodine, Zovirax, Motrin, Premarin, Estrace, Estraderm patch, Vicodin, Lorcet, Questran, Climara, Cytotec, Prilosec, Prozac, Lasix, Toprol, Prednisone, and Claritan. Also, many series of antibiotics, as well as other hormones and cortisone treatments have been prescribed. Some of these helped me for a time. Others did more harm than good. I repeatedly told doctors that the anti-inflammatory drugs did not help the FMS; all they did was cause digestive problems.

PAIN

HOW does one describe the pain? I have never been more totally aware than I am right now, sitting here in front of my computer, of how difficult it is to describe on paper a condition as painful and confusing as the pain of fibromyalgia.

The search for relief from pain is like being lost on a road trip in unfamiliar territory. It is a very dark night; you are going to a place that you have never seen before. You end up on a very dark and lonely road with no signs, no clues, to help you figure out where you are. You finally see a road sign and you think you know where to turn. Then it starts pouring down rain, and you can barely see the road or the turn, and you feel hopeless. Then you see the road to turn on, and you turn, and guess what! It is the wrong road! Your heart is pounding and you are searching for a way out and you get lost further and further—to the point that you think you may be lost forever. You become desperate. I have been on this trip many, many times.

Fibromyalgia pain is not usually apparent to others, and this fact can have very negative effects on the sufferer. These phantom symtoms can cause some inexperienced people to question the reality of FMS and the associated pain. This doubt further isolates the sufferer. It can even cause feelings of guilt in the sufferer, since she (or he) may find herself (himself) defending the pain—maybe even feeling a need to prove it. This is a frustrating and a contradictory feeling. I am sure that you have had people tell you that you don't even look sick. This has happened to me many times. At that precise moment, you may have been wondering how you were going to get through the next few minutes of pain.

I don't think anyone, unless they have lived through it, could fully understand the devastation caused by chronic pain from the top of your head to the tips of your toes and to every part of your life. FMS victims suffer chronic and acute pain for years and years, search ing and searching for any kind of relief. The pain can flare up in a matter of minutes; these flare-ups are a dreaded part of life for the fibromite.

So, let me try to offer a description of the various pains I have experienced in FMS. Chronic pain is pain that usually has a slow onset and lasts for years. (I had chronic leg and jaw pain for over twelve years.) Acute pain has a quick onset and runs a short course (migraines). Some of the pain was localized, but more often it was felt as general pain all over the body. There were arthritic-type pains where the muscles became tight and achy and the joints felt stiff and sore. Headaches were very common and usually led to total body pain. The total body pains sometimes felt achy the way an earache or toothache feels—hot burning sensations along with a feeling that your muscles may explode (unlike the arthritic-type pain). I have been stiff and hardly able to walk. At times, I have just felt sore—as though having been run over by an eighteen wheeler. Sometimes I could hardly stand for clothes to touch me. (Needless to say, physical intimacy was seriously hampered.) I had one or more of these at once and sometimes all of them together.

I lived in chronic pain for over a decade. The first almost appropriate diagnosis for part of my pain was the TMJ, which I believe now was really pain caused from FMS. I had acute flare-ups of pain throughout this time which would occur in a matter of minutes and last what seemed to be forever. Flare-ups could be caused by various situations—lack of sleep, weather conditions, caffeine intake, too much walking or other over exertion or exercise, wearing the wrong kind of shoes, or simply sitting in one position too long. Also, steroid injections caused hormone imbalances and induced flare-ups. On some occasions I have had only back pain or leg pain, but most of the time it was total body pain. Headaches and pressure in my head became part of my daily life.

Foods—so many foods—invited all kinds of pain and adverse effects. Orange juice caused arthritic-type pain. Caffeine gave me irregular heartbeats and leg pain. The day after drinking caffeine, I would notice knots in my left shoulder because, I later found out, caffeine causes waste deposits in the muscles. Irritable bowel syndrome along with muscle pain resulted when I drank milk. Prepared meats, cheeses, and processed foods gave me headaches. Chinese food, MSG, gave me migraines. Sometimes, I reacted badly to wheat and corn products. Too many sweets could result in yeast infections.

Sometimes stress related issues might cause me to get overly emotional and cause pain, headaches, and digestive problems. When my children were younger, I can remember that getting upset with them would instantly cause me to start hurting.

If I cooked a meal, I could not chop up my seasonings with a knife or stand up too long because the pain would become unbearable. I couldn't mop my floors anymore. If I had a lot of paperwork to do, I would end up with a migraine. Chewing hard foods or eating something to require the jaw to pull (like pizza) might cause headaches or muscle pain in the jaw or neck. Sometimes I could be lying in bed, and if my husband just leaned his leg on my body, I would be in intense pain and feel like my legs were going to explode. I was very sensitive to the weather. I could (and still can) often out-perform the weather man and tell my husband when it was going to rain or when a cold front was coming in.

I knew there had to be some information that could help me break this terrible pain cycle. It was a "drive-you-crazy" situation. Regardless of the reason, the pain was very intense and very real. It did not go away easily, if at all, even though I was using different types of pain medications, muscle relaxants, and antidepressants. That changed when I began my natural hormone replacement therapy and stopped using synthetic hormones. The pain difference was like night and day. This made me realize that many of the therapies I had been using were less effective because my hormones were not in balance.

CHAPTER TWO

HORMONES

Versus

HORROR MOANS

DEFINITION AND ROLES

HORROR MOANS! I coined this term when I realized that it described the feelings that I have had for so many years. However, I can happily report that as I have learned to control my pain and to *TAME THOSE HORROR MOANS,* my mind and body have gradually been able to change them back into hormones—the chemicals that, when in balance, can help the body.

Few people, including myself, really understand what they are dealing with when it comes to hormones; this pertains to the medical community, too. To be sure, there have been hormone studies over the years, but they have barely scratched the surface. This is still a relatively unexplored topic in medical science. However, the medical community is slowly beginning to recognize, accept, and discuss the possibility of differences between hormones made by the human body and hormones made from horse urine. This tardiness is because the medical profession follows the lead of the pharmaceutical companies when it comes to medications. In an interview concerning hormone replacement therapy (HRT) in *the International Journal of Pharmaceutical Compounding* (Vol. 2, No. 1, Jan./Feb. 1998), Dr. Christiane Northrup stated that there are more studies on "synthetic" hormones than on "bioidentical" ones because the pharmaceutical companies cannot patent the bioidentical ones. The companies are therefore strongly motivated in favor of the synthetic hormones. In *What Your Doctor May* Not *Tell You About Menopause* (John R. Lee, M.D., and Virginia Hopkins, 1996), the same argument is made.

So what are hormones? I've studied them so much that I think I could pass an exam on them—well, at least on estrogen and progesterone. And there is so very much more to learn. But for a generally accepted definition, we can understand that they are chemical messengers that are made in the endocrine glands such as the pituitary, thyroid, parathyroids, pancreas, adrenals, ovaries, and testes. Also, they may be produced in the pineal and thymus glands, the stomach, the small intestine, and the kidneys. *What Your Doctor May* Not *Tell You About Premenopause* says that some hormones are also made in the fat cells (John R. Lee, M.D., Jesse Hanley, M.D., and Virginia Hopkins, 1999). The blood carries hormones throughout the body to receptor sites on the cells where they are needed. Hormones are involved in all body systems. One can only imagine what a vital role these hormones play in our daily lives.

Production of hormones in the body depends on chemical reactions from chemicals supplied by the diet. A recent statement about this connection of diet and hormones came from the Health Network, "Ask the Family Doctor Show." Dr. Walt Larimore's guest was Dr. James Hughes from the Hilton Head Center for Longevity who stated, "Every time you eat, it's a hormonal event."

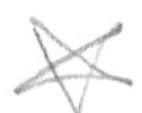

Making hormones correctly and delivering them efficiently for the body's use is a very complex process. If we get the correct proportions of correct nutrients—vitamins, minerals, various other chemicals—for correct chemical reactions in the body, then the result is a contented body which is unaware of the processes going on inside. If, however, the body does not produce enough, or produces too much of a hormone, then we suffer a hormonal imbalance and this can make us painfully aware of body processes.

Hormone imbalances can lead to many health problems, sometimes very serious ones. There are many steps in the process where things can go wrong. As we have said, this can start with what goes into the body. To paraphrase Dr. Lee, toxins enter the body through the mouth, through the airways, or through the skin. Toxins from hazardous chemicals affect hormone balance. But also, bad foods (such as meat from hormone-fed animals) as well as incorrect proportions of good foods can impact hormone balance. Furthermore, some skin preparations, and other substances can disturb natural processes and hormones. (Lee, Hanley, and Hopkins, 1999)

An interesting result of being a fibromite is that now I read everything that comes my way concerning FMS or hormones. I read pamphets in doctors' offices, books, newsletters, newspapers, and more. From reading, I have noticed any number of conditions that improve during pregnancy. Even psoriasis. The authors rarely state that the reason for the improvement may be hormones. It almost seems that the subject is being purposely avoided. There was a tidbit in the December 1999 issue of Arthritis Health Monitor, a pamphelt from a doctor's office. It included a short piece about rheumatoid arthritis easing off during pregnancy in perhaps two thirds of the women studied. The relief ended after delivery. The changes could not be attributed to treatment or to lack of treatment. The final question asked what could have caused the changes. Their answer was that they did not know. My past experiences tell me that there is a hormone imbalance pattern here.

News about foods that have been altered (hormones or genes) and news about environmental effects on human health is increasingly featured on national news programs as well in local news. More doctors writing health books are asserting these connections. Scientific research will prove that these environmental issues are key elements in human hormone balance and in many other health issues. Recent news items reported that major food companies like Gerber, McDonalds, and Frito Lay have rejected altered foods for their products. Europeans have long been on the bandwagon about food sources; they refuse to buy some American foods.

BIOIDENTICAL VERSUS CONVENTIONAL HORMONES

The natural, or bioidentical, hormones made a big difference in my pain experience. So, what are bioidentical hormones, and how are they different from the hormones commonly prescribed? For this summary, I will again take you to the discussions in *What Your Doctor May Not Tell You about Premenopause* (Lee, Hanley, Hopkins, 1999). Page references in this section refer to this book. Dr. Lee and co-authors give a very complete and easily understood explanation. Also read *What Your Doctor May Not Tell You about Menopause* (1996). I strongly urge any person who has hormones in her (or his) body to get one of these books.

There are several terms to understand in this discussion. Bioidentical hormones have the exact same molecular structure as do the hormones produced by the human body. This is true for the estrogens as well as for progesterone. Non-bioidentical hormones have molecular structures that are similar to—but not exactly like—the hormones produced by the human body. "Progestin" is the term used for non-bioidentical progesterone preparations such as Provera. Progestins are alterations of human progesterone because they have a slightly different molecular structure (p 69-70). Phytohormones (phytoestrogens) are plant compounds that have hormonal effects on the body (p 40); phyto is Greek for plant. Xenohormones (xeno means alien) are harmful compounds that have hormonal effects in the body. These include paint solvents; this reminds me of the "old wives tale" warning mothers-to-be not to paint while pregnant.

For centuries, women all over the world have been eating or ingesting plants to relieve "female" problems; in fact, Asian women are known to have fewer "female" problems than do American women because their diets are rich in soy. The Mexican Wild Yam is one of the most popular supplements in our country right now because it is known to have hormonal effects. There are many others with similar qualities. These plants help women to relieve problems with menstrual cycles, premenstrual syndrome, and menopause. Such plants contain phytoestrogens or phytohormones. These plant "estrogens" are much weaker than human estrogens. In fact, phytoestrogens are not really true hormones. They are plant chemicals that have estrogenic or hormonal effects on the body. They attach to the body's estrogen receptors just like the estrogen produced in the body does. By taking up receptor sites, they can have mild positive estrogenic effects and can protect the body from xenohormones (p 37).

Dr. Lee explains that chemicals from phytohormonal plants can be easily altered in the laboratory and synthesized into real hormones. They then become chemical molecules that are exactly like the hormone molecules made by the human body. These are true estrogens and progesterone. These new estrogens are much stronger than the natural plant chemicals, the phytoestrogens, so they are only available by prescription from the doctor. Natural progesterone, however, can be found over-the-counter in pharmacies and in health food stores. Bioidentical or "natural" hormones are much safer than the conjugated estrogens and progestins that I was taking before.

The production or synthesizing of *NATURAL* versus the production or synthesizing of *SYNTHETIC* hormones needs to be understood. It is a confusing issue. The pharmaceuticals say one thing; the "naturalists" say another. The terms get thrown around every which way. That is why in this book we choose to use the terms bioidentical and non-bioidentical for the most part. Many doctors are unfamiliar with the issue, and that can cause you problems if you do not understand the difference yourself.

First, let's examine the production of progesterone. Bioidentical progesterone and non-bioidentical progestins are both produced (synthesized) from the same plants (the wild yam or other similar plants). Therefore, they can both be described as synthetic—they are synthesized. On the other hand, they can both be called *natural* because both are produced from natural plant sources. The important difference is that the bioidentical progesterone is synthesized to have exactly the same chemical or molecular structure as the progesterone that is produced by your own body, whereas the progestins are not (Lee, Hanley, Hopkins, 1999).

So, you can choose to take progesterone (bioidentical), which is the one that is natural to the human body with no known negative side effects if used in physiologic doses (same amount as the body should make-p 80). Lee explains that it does, however, **offer some good effects** according to scientific studies. Some of the most notable ones are: **protects against fibrocystic breasts, is a natural diuretic, helps to use fat for energy, helps thyroid action, aids in blood clotting and blood sugar functions, protects against some cancers and against osteoporosis.** (Lee, Hopkins, ...*Menopause* p72)

Or you can choose to take a **progestin, like Provera,** which is not real progesterone, but is a substance with a similar, but not the same, molecular structure. It has some possible, **serious side effects.** These include **increased risk of birth defects, cancer, vision problems, menstrual irregularities, depression, fluid retention, and a host of others** (pp. 86-88 in the Lee, Hopkins book).

The production of estrogen presents a similar story according to the Dr. Lee books. Bioidentical estrogens—there are several—are synthesized from plants. However, the *non*-bioidentical estrogens such as Premarin contain estrogens from the urine of pregnant mares as well as human estrogens. Both sources—plants and horse urine—are considered natural sources and this is the cause of the confusion. The pharmaceutical industry, and therefore many doctors, considers Premarin to be a *natural* hormone product, but it is not natural to humans.

The very important lesson here is that you must be very clear and descriptive when you talk to your doctor about natural hormones. Both of you may use the term *natural hormones* while each of you is discussing a different product. This actually happened to me and this experience is told in the section titled "My Journey to Natural Hormones."

Of special interest is that research on hormones is increasing and is beginning to confirm what some women and doctors already believe—that bioidentical and non-bioidentical hormones act very differently in the human body. Moreover, there are medical consequences, especially for women, for not understanding these differences. Dr. Christiane Northrup is a holistic obstetrician-gynecologist who edits the newsletter *Health Wisdom for Women, (she also* authored *Women's Bodies, Women's Wisdom).* In an article about hormone replacement, she quoted Dr. David Zava, Ph.D., a 20-year researcher and the director of Aaron Labs in San Leandro, CA.; Zava says that both progesterone and progestin are metabolized in the body to produce "breakdown" or "daughter" products. The "metabolic daughter compounds" produced in the body from bioidentical hormones are different from those produced from "synthetic" hormones. The "daughter" compounds from progestins can cause negative side effects. She also cites Joel Hargrove, M.D., director of the Menopause Center at Vanderbilt University. Hargrove stated that non-bioidentical estrogen (like Premarin) metabolizes to form breakdown products that are stronger than the original estrogens. Therefore, the effects of estrogen are prolonged in the body, rather than clearing out, as intended by nature. The prolonged effect of estrogen is a cancer risk. *(International Journal of Pharmaceutical Compounding, Jan/Feb, 1998).*

COMPOUNDING PHARMACY

I use hormones which are compounded locally by compounding pharmacist Peter Wolfe, Jr., R.PH. of Total Pharmacy Services, Inc. in Houma, Louisiana. He and his associates have been very patient and helpful to me in my trials with bioidentical hormone therapy. They have answered thousands of my questions.

Compounding pharmacists are compared to pharmacists as they used to be in the old days. Then, the pharmacist actually mixed medical preparations rather than buying them already prepared. The already-prepared formulas are good in that they avoid some amount of human error in the preparation. But, there is still a need for the unique expertise of compounding pharmacists. Wolfe explains that his pharmacy fills a niche that the normal pharmacies tend to avoid because of the specialized (and expensive) equipment needed to do this work properly. Moreover, the work is very time consuming and requires additional training.

In the case of the progesterone that I use, the compounding pharmacy buys the product already synthesized from the natural plant by a larger lab. It carries the label USP (United States Pharmacopeia). This label indicates that the product meets the governmental standards required for "pharmaceutical grade" products. The pharmacist can then mix it with other substances as needed and as directed by the doctor.

Compounding prescriptions have several advantages. Besides the value of using bioidentical hormones, there is also the advantage of mixing various pharmaceuticals for the unique needs of the patient. The doctor may want the patient to have one estrogen, but not the others. Or he may want to dictate how much of each of the estrogens to give to the patient. The compounding pharmacist can mix these to the doctors specifications.

Natural, compounded hormones can be produced in several forms—biestrogen capsules, triestrogen capsules, creams, or suppositories—which permits different personal preferences to be accommodated. They can be compounded in varying strengths and combinations and tailored to the individual, although there are some formulas that have become somewhat standard as a starting point for prescription.

The compounded hormones are very easy to adjust by the patient, by the doctor, or by the compounding pharmacist. This, to me, is a very important consideration. Every person's medication needs are unique, just as their appetite and nutrient needs are unique. Even people with the same disease, or imbalance, need different levels of treatment. I was able to work with the pharmacist to make minute changes in the strength of the prescription. I prefer creams because it is so easy to increase or decrease the dosage; capsules do not offer this flexibility. The point is that different personal preferences or needs can be accommodated.

MY JOURNEY TO NATURAL HORMONES

At about thirteen years of age I began having menstrual cycles. It was a difficult time for me. Each month I would lie in bed in extreme pain before and during the menstrual period. This went on until I was married. My first baby was born about a year after I married, and I had another baby about three years later. I can honestly say I felt my best when I was pregnant. What was so different about pregnancy? I think my hormones had corrected themselves, and that is why I felt so healthy and energetic.

During the next several years, I took birth control pills, up to the time of my hysterectomy. I had migraines every month either before or during my period. The headaches were intense enough to interrupt my life. I had TMJ surgery during this time. Also, I began to have more symptoms of fibromyalgia, including digestive problems, body aches, and sleep problems. This was diagnosed as fibrocitis; I thus began the long-term use of anti-inflammatory medications. I began having pelvic pain caused by endometriosis, fibroid tumors, and prolapsed uterus. These symptoms later resulted in a complete hysterectomy. After the hysterectomy I began hormone injections; they were bad for me, but the experience did lead me into the search that would finally find my answer.

When taking the hormone injections after the hysterectomy, I would hurt badly for about the first six or seven days after the shot; I now know this was an FMS flare-up. Then it would let up for about a week. After this week, and until the next injection, I would start to feel badly, having FMS symptoms, as well as migraines, hot flashes, and other PMS symptoms. The injections were supposed to last a month but they lasted only two weeks at most. I was not allowed another shot until at least three weeks had passed, so for one week my suffering was worse than usual. My whole existence was just eating, sleeping, and suffering. It was a miserable experience. I finally switched to a hormone patch with some degree of relief except that the migraines were worse.

The hysterectomy failed to cure the symptoms I had expected it to. About this time, I became keenly aware when others discussed fibromyalgia or hysterectomies. I started contacting as many of these women as I could, to see if we had any similarities. Many of the women had undergone hysterectomies or were menopausal or were on some type of conventional hormone or thyroid medications. This really made me think about my situation. My hysterectomy (Dec. 1996) had put me into surgical menopause and I was on hormone treatments.

The time for a mammogram came, and I went to a conventional doctor. One problem that had not abated since the hysterectomy was loss of libido, so I mentioned this to the doctor. He was sure that I needed testosterone: he gave me an injection of estrogen and testosterone together. The shot did nothing for the libido problem; he prescribed a testosterone pill. I took it for only three days because it caused terrible migraines. I felt miserable for three weeks. At the next appointment, the doctor gave me a double injection of estrogen and testosterone. What a bad mistake! And, how I did pay for that mistake! That very night I had the worst fibromyalgia symptoms of my entire life, including large knots in my legs. I had other sorts of leg pains; it felt like my legs would explode. I had bad joint aches, severe lower back pain, and migraines. I also had digestive problems including heartburn, diarrhea, and irritable bowel. I couldn't sleep. I had blurred vision and heart palpitations. As the shot effects wore off, after about two weeks, the fibromyalgia symptoms abated. I returned one more time, and that time the doctor informed me that he feared that my endometriosis had returned--I thought that was impossible because both ovaries had been removed in the hysterectomy.

The pain from the hormone shot indicated to me that my suspicions of a connection between fibromyalgia and hormones must be right. At that point, I knew two things---one, that I needed hormones to avoid the post-hysterectomy menopausal symptoms, and second, that the hormone injections were causing the fibromyalgia flare-ups. Coincidentally, I stumbled on *Smart Medicine for Menopause* by Sandra Cabot, M.D. The book addressed several of my problems. For one thing, she pointed out that:

> Endometriosis can be reactivated by estrogen replacement unless sufficient progesterone is taken to balance the estrogen therapy. Women with a past history of endometriosis (whether they have had a hysterectomy or not) should take low-dose progesterone tablets continually along with estrogen (p. 59)

Her book led me to the health food store where I bought some progesterone cream. I also started using the Climara hormone patch again because Cabot said that it contained a natural form of estrogen (estradiol). Again, the Climara patch gave me migraine headaches. I later learned that although Estradiol is a natural hormone, it is the strongest one of the estrogen complex.

I first started taking natural-to-the-human-body or bioidentical hormones in September of 1998. I was helped and supervised by a doctor of integrative medicine. I became familiar with the term "integrative medicine" when the sales person in the health food store gave me a pamphlet on it. Integrative doctors use both conventional and alternative methods and treatments. I went to her looking for a better post-hysterectomy hormone treatment—one that would not cause migraine headaches as the "patch" treatments did.

After various prescriptions failed, the integrative doctor gave me estrogen, in the form of Tri-Est, and a 10% progesterone gel. The amount of Tri-Est was too much—the left side of my neck became stiff (like a crick) every morning and I suffered hot flashes. I experimented with the amount of cream, according to the Cabot book suggestions. I did manage to eliminate the stiff neck, but the hot flashes persisted. I was beginning to feel more comfortable, and now I could hope for even better results if I could find the right formula.

I was on the "natural" or bioidentical hormones for about six weeks. Even my fibromyalgia leg pain got better, but because I was so focused on migraines, endometriosis pain, and menopausal symptoms, I still did not associate the effects of the *bioidentical/natural form* of the hormones and the fibromyalgia pain.

THEN, the doctor moved away leaving me to find another doctor; this was a very depressing turn of events. It was the first of several events that would finally show me the certain difference between the conventional hormones and the bioidentical hormones and the amazing different effects that each had on my body.

The feeling that I was on the right track was good, but I needed a doctor's help to monitor and supervise the treatments. I called another doctor who had been highly recommended. Before making an appointment I asked if she prescribed "natural" hormones. The receptionist checked with the doctor and told me that she did. However, as I have pointed out, the word "natural" means different things to different people. The doctor prescribed Premarin (6.75 mg.), promising me that, " it *is* natural." I reluctantly agreed since I was not yet comfortable with my own knowledge about which hormones are "natural".

After two weeks on Premarin, I experienced another FMS flare-up. I stopped the hormones, and that action alone helped somewhat. I looked up Premarin in *Screaming to Be Heard* by Elizabeth Lee Vliet, M.D., a book that my neurologist suggested. What I read made me realize that Premarin was not a product that I thought of as natural.

I still needed a doctor who would help me with the natural hormones. Dr. John Milek had been compassionate, understanding, and easy to talk to before; by now he was back on my insurance plan, so I went back to him. He helped me restart and adjust the dosages of the bioidentical hormones—the program I am following now. I began to feel better right away, and by the end of three months the fibromyalgia symptoms had abated. Also, the menopausal symptoms and the migraines were under control.

I was so elated that I started this book.

Can you draw your own conclusions as I did? Make the connection!

My FMS Symptoms:	Some Hormonal Imbalance Symptoms:
1. Fatigue	1. Fatigue
2. Muscle pain	2. Muscle pain
3. Joint pain	3. Joint pain
4. Low libido	4. Low libido
5. Digestive problems	5. Digestive problems
6. Anxiety	6. Anxiety
7. Depression	7. Depression
8. Heart palpitations	8. Heart palpitations
9. Migraines	9. Migraines
10. Vaginal Dryness	10. Vaginal Dryness
11. Poor memory	11. Poor memory
12. Frequent urination	12. Frequent urination
13. Poor sleep	13. Poor sleep
14. Hot flashes	14. Hot flashes
15. Facial hair	15. Facial hair
16. Headaches	16. Headaches

CHAPTER THREE

THE VICTORY PLAN

MY PERSONAL Rx

INTRODUCTION

The best chapter!!! It is so fantastic to be able to share with you the strategies and therapies that have boosted me up. It is absolutely thrilling to share the positive news about bioidentical hormones and the almost total relief from FMS that they gave me. It is important to tell you how I adapted treatments to my own use, so that you will not reject them at the first sign of failure. That is a real temptation to FMS sufferers, most of whom have had many experiences with dead-end therapies. But quick rejection can prove to be shortsighted. Follow me through the treatments I experienced and see if any of them might be of help to your situation. Keep in mind that I have been under a doctor's care for most of them. I also get help from various professional therapists, and from pharmacists. I call them often. My advice is not to try new therapies alone. Get competent and caring help.

The main "tools" that I used and still use are discussed in this section. Let me say right here that drinking lots of water all day is so important that is has been almost like one of the treatments or therapies. All of the therapists and chiropractors recommended lots of water to eliminate toxins. Also, it is important to drink lots of water, about 16 to 24 ounces, within an hour after massage therapy. Drinking adequate amounts of water helps to reduce or prevent migraines or tight muscles.

I have tried other therapies to improve my condition; they include meditation, visualization, relaxation tapes, reflexology and Reiki. All of them seemed to help some. I still use the meditation, and sometimes the visualization, for any kind of pain. Few people are familiar with reflexology and Reiki. According to the *Reader's Digest Guide to Natural Medicine* (1994), reflexology is a form of foot and hand pressure massage. Reiki is a therapy to relieve energy blockages in the body. Reiki helped a little more. Although reflex ology and Reiki were somewhat less effective than other therapies, I would use them again because they feel good and are great tools for relaxation.

Supplementing the diet with nutrients is important. Without adequate vitamins, minerals, and other nutritional supplements, the body cannot overcome maladies and function correctly. It is becoming ever more apparent that nutritional supplementation is necessary for the stressful, contaminated, and medicated lives we live. There are medical tests that can determine which nutrients are deficient in a person's body, and learning about nutrition is easier now with all the books and radio and television shows that teach which nutrients to use for which problems as well as which ones to avoid in certain situations. You are what you eat.

CHOOSING THE TEAM

Remember that you are the captain. The team is crucial to the achievement of success against FMS. The team should include a wonderful, compassionate doctor as coach, a pharmacist, other professionals, and your family. I thank God that I have such a loving husband and children. My mother and siblings have been very caring and supportive. Friends and coworkers can also be wonderful and helpful allies. I will always be grateful to those of my family, friends, and co-workers who have understood and helped me.

Choosing the team can be challenging. The family is already chosen; some members may be more supportive than others, but that is true in any situation and in any family. Choosing the friends to help requires an understanding of personalities and their abilities to support you. The pharmacist should be someone who will answer questions about medications very willingly and thoroughly. The doctor may be the hardest to choose. A doctor who believes that fibromyalgia is a disease is of utmost importance; it is hard to believe how many still do not. Moreover, he should be willing to work with you in trying various treatments and medications; as the coach of your team, he should be willing to let you call some of the plays. If he cannot, or will not, work with you, then it is better to find another doctor who can and will do so.

It is extremely important to communicate well with the team, and it is something that can be learned and constantly improved. It takes work and patience on the part of the already fragile fibromite, but learning effective communication is worth the effort. You do not have to bear everything in silence; sheer silence can isolate you from people who might help. I had to learn to express my pain and my feelings. This was not easy, especially when I perceived that others thought I was exaggerating or imagining the pain. It has become easier now that the medical community acknowledges the disease.

Even a master communicator may find it hard to convey the confusing plight of FMS. It was very hard for me to remember that if others (team members or not) did not suffer chronic pain themselves, they probably did not have the knowledge to fully appreciate my situation. It is stressful when someone very close to you cannot understand your pain and frustration. Some of my co-workers never did acknowledge my suffering. It seemed like they thought it was something to joke about. My ability to accept this lack of understanding and to learn to deal with it was an important lesson and stress reducer for me. It motivated me to fend for myself, and that is when I began to make real progress.

STAYING COMFORTABLE

It is important as a fibromite to be kind to your body. There are several strategies that I use to do this. These are the little things you can do, but they can help a lot.

Posture is very important. I learned to sit or stand straight. I try to keep my spine aligned properly no matter what the activity.

When sitting for longer periods, I use either the magnet pads or one of the various types of pillow designed especially to prevent body pain. Footstools, with or without magnets, as well as other posture aids can help avoid pain when you have to sit for a long while.

Riding in a car for more than an hour can be uncomfortable, so I make it a habit to get out and walk around for a few minutes every once in a while. There are stretches (see pictures) you can do in the car.

Standing still for long periods, for example at parties or business meetings, is really hard on me. I started wearing low, thick cushioned shoes. I constantly shift weight from side to side and change general body position. And, if I can, I sit down for just one or two minutes every once in a while, perhaps every forty-five minutes. This will usually stop the pain from developing further, or it may at least take the edge off of the already present pain.

These tactics are still important to me. However, now that I am using the bioidentical hormones rather than the synthetic ones, I can ride in a car without stopping as often and I have less pain when sitting or standing for long periods.

SLEEP

Sleep is a very important factor in fibromyalgia. Failure to get adequate sleep will cause the fibromite to suffer the next day and the pain usually will be worse than usual.

During sleep the body rejuvenates itself. Serotonin is replenished during deep (level four) sleep. Many fibromites fail to reach this deep level of sleep, and that is why doctors so often prescribe sleep medication, as well as antidepressants, for them. I was on Elavil before I started using the bioidentical hormones, and it did help me sleep deeply. But the problem with the Elavil was that it made me want to sleep most of the next day, even if I took it early the evening before.

Exercise is important to me as a sleep aid. When I exercise routinely, I sleep better, and therefore I wake up feeling much more refreshed. Magnet pads are a super sleep aid as well; they are described in detail in another section.

A superior mattress is very crucial for good sleep. It has been said that FMS patients have the most comfortable beds in the world. Any money spent for a good mattress is valid; think of it as preventing the pain and dollars of a doctor visit. Also, I use an "egg-crate" pad on my bed, a strategy I learned from the hospital. Some hospitals have started using air mattresses and they are also very comfortable. Hotel beds can cause problems for the fibromite. Earlier on, if we stayed in a hotel, I would wake up with more than usual pain, so I started sleeping on the magnet seat pad from the car, and this made a significant difference.

Natural hormone therapy has corrected most of my sleep problems. Hormones have a natural antidepressant effect. I have been able to discontinue using the Elavil and I am sleeping deeper than ever before. I no longer wake up at every slight noise; this resolves a lifelong problem. My nightmares are gone. My sleep is so much improved that I was motivated, after years of dreading mornings, to start a routine by setting my clock at the same hour every morning, and moving the hour earlier little by little. I gradually started waking up before the alarm, with the energy and desire to get up *now* rather than wanting to sleep all day like before. The fibrofog was gone.

TRANSCUTANEOUS ELECTRICAL NERVE STIMULATION—TENS

The TENS unit has been familiar to athletes for years. It is a small electronic device designed to provide relief from pain. Athletes use it to relieve the pain of overworked muscles. Others use it for different pains—acute, chronic, or post-operative. Postoperative patients have been known to use less pain medication with the help of the TENS unit. Some chiropractors use them to help patients relax and thus promote easier and more complete spinal adjustment.

The TENS unit works by sending out electrical current which travels under the skin stimulating nerve fibers; this blocks the pain signals traveling along the nerves prohibiting them from reaching the brain. The unit offers controls so that the patient can change the pattern or the strength of the electrical current.

I realized that acute pain responded best to this electrical therapy; chronic pain, somewhat less effectively. I came to depend on it especially if I experienced a pain flare-up. In fact, using this therapy produced positive results often enough that I used it periodically for a number of years.

There are several types of TENS units. I have used two of them. One unit employs one to four small, sticky electrodes to be placed at various points of the body to deliver the current. This is the one I have used for years. It is convenient in that it can be worn under clothing while you work. I would use two or four electrodes depending on the space between the pain points; if only arm/neck area or only leg/back/pelvic area hurt, I used only two electrodes; if it all hurt, then I used all four electrodes. I placed two electrodes on the upper back part of the hips for lower body region. For upper body region, I placed them slightly above and inside the shoulder blades.

However, there are some drawbacks to consider. In my experience, prolonged use of the electrode-type TENS unit would cause a burning pain different from the ones I was trying to alleviate. I could sometimes wear it for up to twelve hours and gain relief, but its use for longer periods became counter-productive. Wearing it only one or two hours a day for several days worked better. Moreover, I found another problem—after using the unit four to five times a week for about eight months, it became less effective. After this long period, the nervous system tends to ignore the electrical impulses, and increasingly higher settings are needed to resolve pain. Increasing the strength and changing the patterns of current helped for a while, but my body continued to adapt to the changed settings. I asked around and found that this is rather common. The lesson is to use the unit very sporadically. A final warning is for those with pacemakers; they should never use this therapy.

The small gun type of TENS is the other one I used. It allowed me to stimulate particular trigger points. This is helpful because when an area hurts, the stimulus of the pain can be a trigger point that is completely removed from the hurting area. For example, I might experience pain in the pelvic area, and the site to stimulate would be a trigger point in the lower back. Or, I could have hand or arm pain coming from a trigger point on the shoulder. This unit beeps as you move it over an area. When the beep gets very high-pitched and fast, a trigger point has been located; you then release the current to that exact point for fifteen to thirty seconds. This can be done more than once, but I did not usually need to do so. Relief from pain would sometimes come within a few minutes, or I would try again to get results. At times, during a bad flare-up, the method did not work at all. Extremely helpful for the success of this unit was the chart showing trigger points and the areas these points could influence; the Starlynl/Copeland book has these charts.

When I discovered magnet therapy, I gave up using TENS therapy for the most part, although I have gone back to it occasionally. I use the TENS unit sometimes if I over exert on some kind of task which causes muscle tension in the neck area or aggravates a TMJ flare-up.

TENS therapy, then, has been quite helpful to me. At that time, any relief at all was worth the time and effort spent learning to adjust it to my unique needs. With it, I could function longer at different tasks. At times I had up to a fifty percent reduction in pain. The therapy allowed me to reduce pain medication while performing physical activities, like walking, done to improve my overall condition. I still recommend it to anyone who is searching for pain relief.

RS-4M MUSCLE STIMULATOR

Many doctors are now prescribing this unit to their patients; it is only available by prescription. My doctor prescribed this stimulator for spasms in my neck and back after I fell. Although I discovered this unit after conquering FMS, it is reportedly very helpful to fibromites, and so I feel it would be beneficial to explain how it works.

The RS-4M stimulator has eight self-adhesive electrode pads to be placed at strategic points on the body, and there are four individually controlled channels for treatment flexibility. Small electrical impulses cause the muscles to contract and relax, just like the muscles do in normal movement. The stimulator focuses on a specific muscle or muscle group, and is used to relax muscle spasms, prevent muscle weakness, and increase range of motion and local blood circulation. Medical studies have shown that therapy that conditions the muscles speeds recovery and increases comfort during rehabilitation.

Because the unit is portable, it can be used anywhere. The user should be sitting, lying down, or in a relaxed position to use it. I use it while watching TV or reading. It is very relaxing. I feel like I've had a massage after using the stimulator.

If you want more information on this therapy, call R. S. Medical, Inc. at (360) 892-0339 or look up the Internet site at www.rsmedical.com.

MAGNETIC THERAPY

This is treatment that utilizes magnets at various points on the body. I use the Nikken brand of magnets, and I salute the Nikken company for a superior product. There are magnets which can be worn on any part of the body and there are magnets designed for specific usage—shoe inserts, necklaces, back belts, massage bars, massaging balls, pillows and mattresses, and more. Magnet treatments are gaining in acceptability as more research seems to substantiate patient-reported effectiveness. They are now often included in "legitimate" discussions on alternative therapy.

I discovered magnet therapy over four years ago. In fact, magnet use was the very first treatment that I found to offer really significant relief to my years and years and years of almost constant pain. It was magnet therapy that soothed my pain like nothing else ever had before. You can't imagine the positive effect that such remarkable physical relief had on my emotions and outlook. This was a breakthrough for me and gave me new hope for finding a more normal life.

Magnets are still a part of my life to this day, and they probably always will be. Using them, I have achieved different levels of relief depending on what type of pain I was having. For example, weather related (TMJ), arthritic, or joint aches respond better than the burning, pressure kind of pain that most FMS patients experience.

My personal use of magnets started with shoe inserts. I started wearing them a little each day and gradually increased the time to about half a day, depending on the amount of time I walked that day. Notably, if I walked all day on the magnets, the pain worsened—the literature on magnets discourages all day use. I usually wore them in shoes that allowed for thick socks because wearing them with thin socks made my feet burn. Thus, wearing the shoe insert magnets reduced the muscle soreness and helped to reduce most of the pelvic pain experienced while trying to function during the day.

Gradually, I started to use more kinds of magnets. The back magnet belt was the one that I used the most, because it treated my most common pain sites. The magnet balls are the most powerful of all the magnets, and are especially effective; I use them to massage or rub the areas that hurt. This method reduces the pain to a level low enough that I can ignore it. In fact, after the massage with magnet balls, I then wear a magnet strip on that same area, and these two procedures together can almost totally eliminate the pain for up to several hours or until I perform another "pain-aggravating" activity. Since my job requires that I travel quite a bit, I use the magnet pad in the car. This helps tremendously because I can sit for longer periods of time and feel very comfortable. In the past, before adding the magnet (and other) strategies, I would have total body pain by bedtime, so I began to sleep on the magnet mattress pad—the same one used by so many sports players. Lying on this pad, I can actually feel a pulling sensation as though it is pulling the pain away. Before I had the mattress, it would take hours to fall asleep even if I took pain medicine. The mattress relieves the pain enough for me to fall asleep normally and to sleep better. However, since finding the bioidentical hormone therapy, I only need the mattress occasionally.

Therapy must be a daily habit with chronic fibromyalgia I have learned. Therefore, my habit was to use the magnets every day, or almost every day, in some manner. Now, though, after over four years of use, I have altered my FMS to the point that I do not have to wear a magnet except for the TMJ problem and the herniated disk problem. When I hurt, I wear a magnet for several hours and that almost always stops the pain until something aggravates the situation enough to restart the pain. If I wake up with pain or if I know that I will be doing paper work or physical activities known to aggravate pain, I use one of the magnets as a preventive measure.

If all of this hasn't convinced you, I will tell you about my uncle. He had back problems for most of his adult life. He had to take medicine every night to be able to go to sleep. Many nights he ended up sleeping on the floor. I bought him a back magnet belt to wear around his waist. He wore it faithfully for about a year, and now he has no more back pain and rarely uses the magnet. In fact, he loaned it to a friend.

The use of magnet therapy, then, has reduced my general pain, on the one-to-ten scale used by so many doctors, from a level of ten to a level of about five, sometimes for hours of time. Moreover, using the magnets allowed me to decrease my pain medicine and still function on a daily basis. Since I achieved significant pain reduction, after so many false hopes, my fibromyalgia depression also improved.

For information on Nikken magnets, call 1-888-2Nikken, or see their web site at www.nikken.com.

EXERCISE

Exercise has finally proven to be very useful in my pain management plan. The worst thing the fibromite can do is just lie around; the muscles suffer more, not less, with too much inactivity. Knowing that exercise stimulates the producton of endorphins that stop pain made me eager to do them. However, learning which exercises to do, how often to do them, and how long to do them was not easy to sort out. Sometimes my pain would be as bad or worse after exercise. I could not tell, early on, if the exercise itself was causing pain, or if it was the FMS. Neither did the doctors know, as the condition was new to them, too; like me they were trying various methods.

Anti-inflammatory or muscle relaxant medications would sometimes mask the pain caused by exercise; I would then not feel the pain until too late and would experience a flare-up. That would prompt the doctor to increase the medicines. It was a vicious cycle.

Upon being diagnosed with FMS, various doctors recommended stretch exercises. Of course they would give me a pat regimen that they gave to all patients—ten of this stretch, ten of that stretch, etc. I tried the recommended stretch exercises with no relief or with bad results. I now know that I was trying too much, too soon. Discouraged, I would avoid the stretches for a while in favor of other forms of exercise—walking, stationary bicycle, chiropractor, etc.

In one of my attempts, I joined a health spa with my family, again in response to advice to exercise. I still believed that if I strengthened my muscles, the daily pain of the FMS would at least be somewhat alleviated. I told the trainer about my fibromyalgia, and he assured me that he had supervised such cases before. He started me out on the treadmill (20-30 min.), the bicycle (15 min.), and the rowing machine (10-min.). In short order I ended up in terrible shape.

Walking, too, has caused me grief. Over the years I have tried the suggested walking programs. I would walk the suggested twenty to thirty minutes and then suffer extreme pain in my legs, back, and pelvic area. Too much walking, or any exercise, caused such pain that I could not sleep at night. The lack of sleep kept my body's chemical balance out of kilter.

I finally did manage to devise exercises for myself that do help. The right exercises done the right way for me are illustrated at the end of this section; they are:

❖ Stretching is the most important one. It can be done anytime, anywhere. Without stretching, I cannot do other exercises without causing pain. Gentle is the key word; always stretch gently. I stretch very often during the day. I stretch when I wake up, after sitting at the desk for a while, after any kind of exercises, or if I feel tension building anywhere in my body. Stretching exercises can help to prevent sore, tight muscle pain very effectively. It also helps somewhat to control joint pain. Daily activities are much more pain free when I remember to stretch often.

❖ Breathing exercises are beneficial to get oxygen to the muscles and to relax muscle tension. Breathe in through the nose—a deep breath that makes your stomach expand; hold the breath a moment; then breathe audibly out through the mouth. An excellent book to use as a breathing guide is Pam Grout's *Jumpstart Your Metabolism.*

❖ Walking, on a treadmill or anywhere, is almost as important as stretching. Walking the treadmill is somewhat more likely than regular walking to cause pain, so extra care is needed. I can walk around the block, if slowly, for thirty minutes; on the treadmill I have only worked up to twenty or thirty minutes. Nevertheless, I prefer the treadmill—it is handy and room temperature is controlled. If I have not walked or exercised for a week or so, then I start my program over at the lowest level and work up to maximum limits. The first day I walk only one minute at a speed of two mph or less on the treadmill, on day two, two minutes, etc. Always after walking, I do just a few gentle stretches—leg, back, whole body. The stretches are crucial to prevent pain! I always maintain a speed low enough that I feel no pain while doing the walking. Grout describes another walking technique—walking with a sip of water in the mouth. The American Indians used this to build stamina. It causes you to improve breathing and to pump oxygen into the body (*Jumpstart your Metabolism*).

- ❖ Water exercises are very beneficial to some fibromites. Most health clubs teach water exercises. Each person needs to find his/her own body tolerances. Exercising in cold water is worse than not exercising at all—it tightens the muscles and causes pain. However, exercising in a heated pool can be as beneficial as walking. Heated pools can be hard to find. No health clubs here had one, so I made arrangements with a local hotel to exercise there.

- ❖ Bicycling is as beneficial as walking for some. As with other exercises, start out slowly. Do not do too much too fast. I had limited luck with bicycling for a time because of other health problems—endometriosis and tilted uterus. I preferred walking during that time. However, after the hysterectomy, bicycling felt beneficial and comfortable again.

The **exercises to avoid**, for me anyway, include weight lifting (even light weights), yoga, stair master, and rowing. I avoid all exercise machines that require push and pull movements (like the rowing machine). Exercise just before bedtime is to be avoided; I exercise in the early morning, in the middle of the day, or in the early evening at least two hours before bedtime for best results.

One very important thing I have learned is when to stop the exercise. If I feel any hint of pain or excess physical stress, I stop the exercise. I wait a day and then start the exercise again at a slower or gentler level. This is very important. For me, overdoing an exercise does more harm than not doing it at all.

With the proper methods, time limits, and intensity, exercise has been very beneficial to me. The exercises that have helped me the most are stretching, walking, and breathing exercises. With regular exercise, at least three to five times a week, I sleep more soundly and minor noises do not wake me. Moreover, I wake up feeling more energetic. Exercise helps to lessen the early-morning "irritable everything" syndrome called fibrofog familiar to so many frbromites.

The
Treadmill and Bicycle
are very beneficial!

I always stretch
Immediately after exercising!

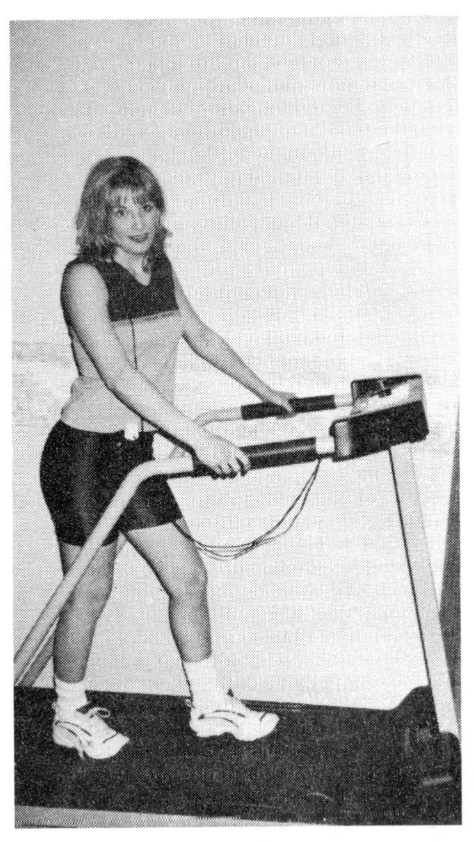

figure: 1

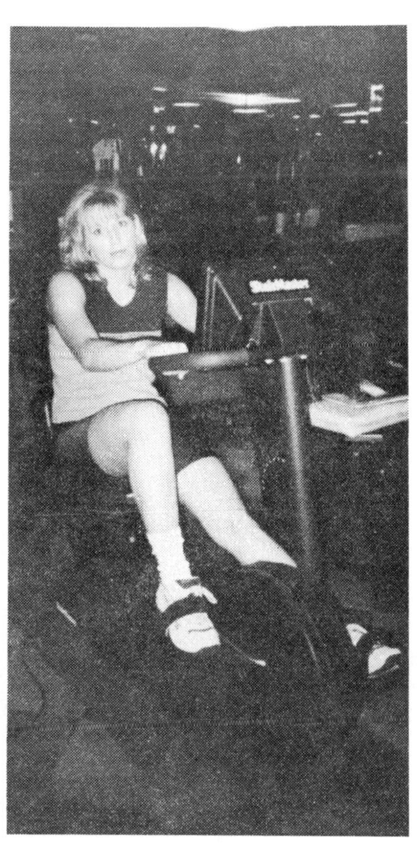

figure: 2

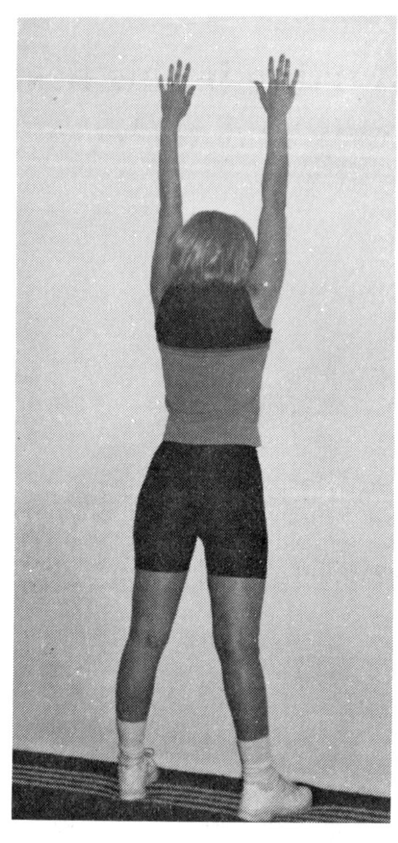

Stretch as high as you can and then relax!

figure 3

Stretch as wide as you can and then relax!

figure 4:

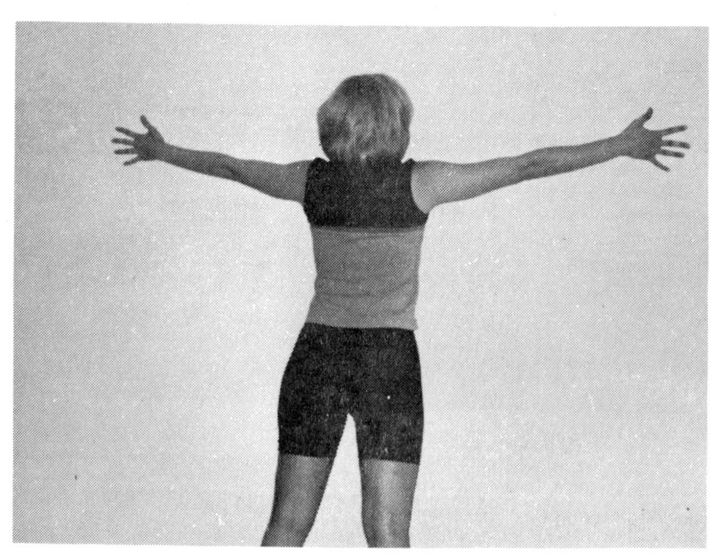

Do the next 3 stretches starting in this first position and come up slowly and arch your back.

figures 5-7:

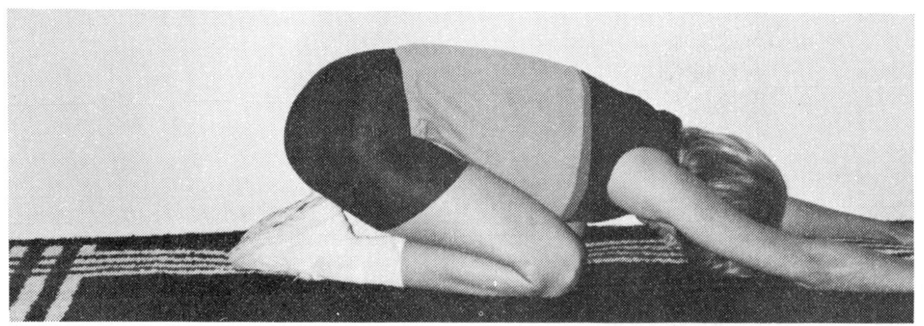

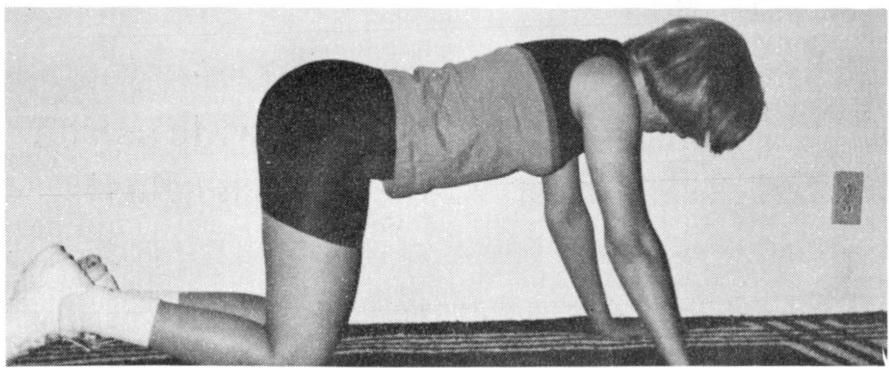

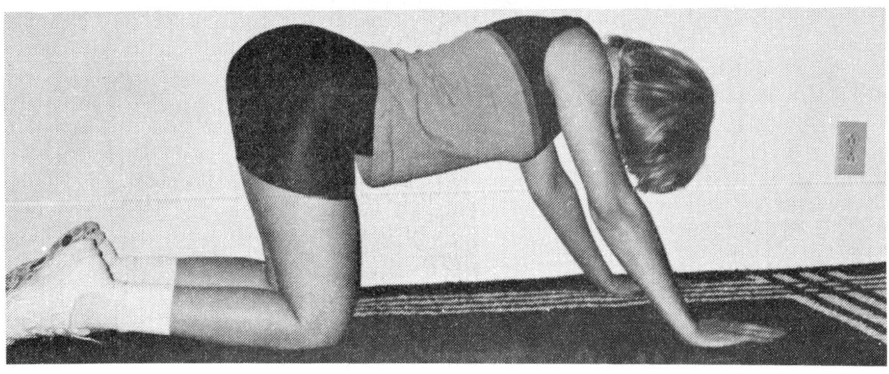

Stretch out each leg and point your toes and then relax

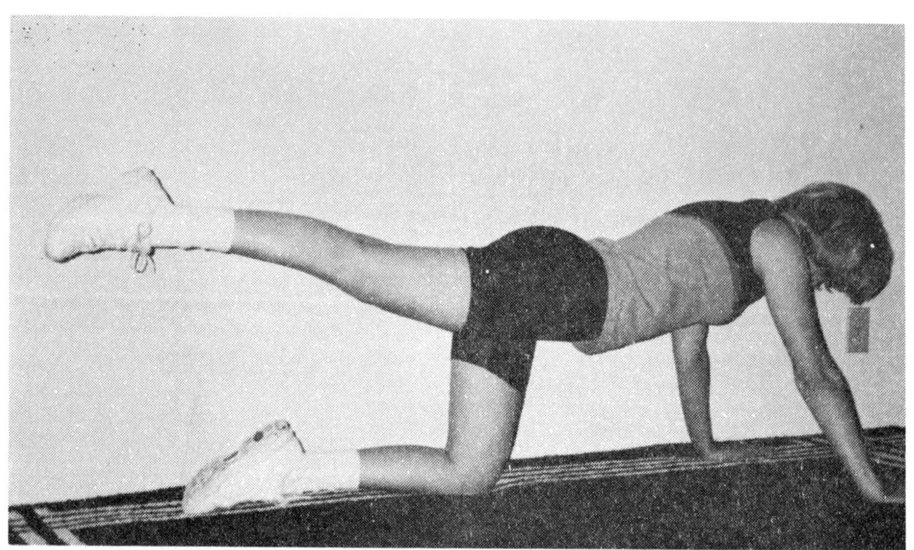

figure: 8

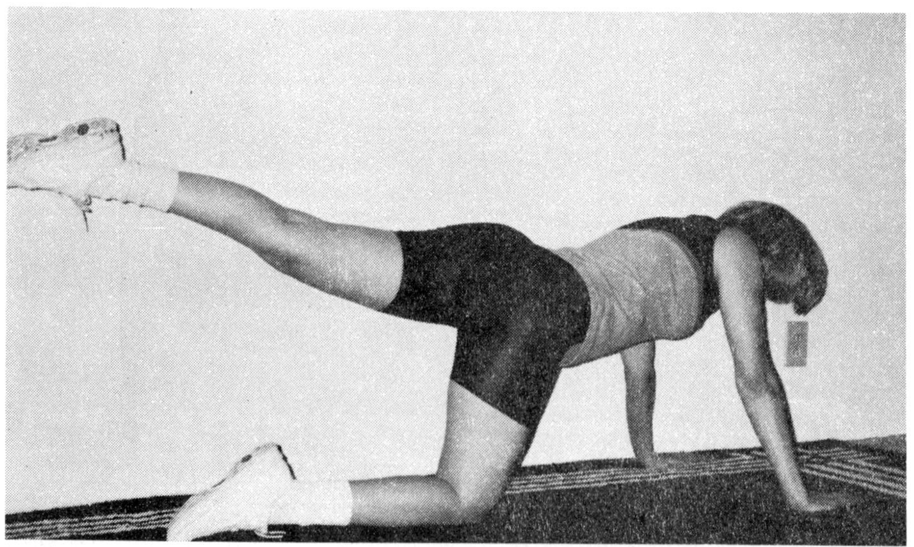

figure: 9:

Sit comfortably & point your toes out and then relax:

figure 10

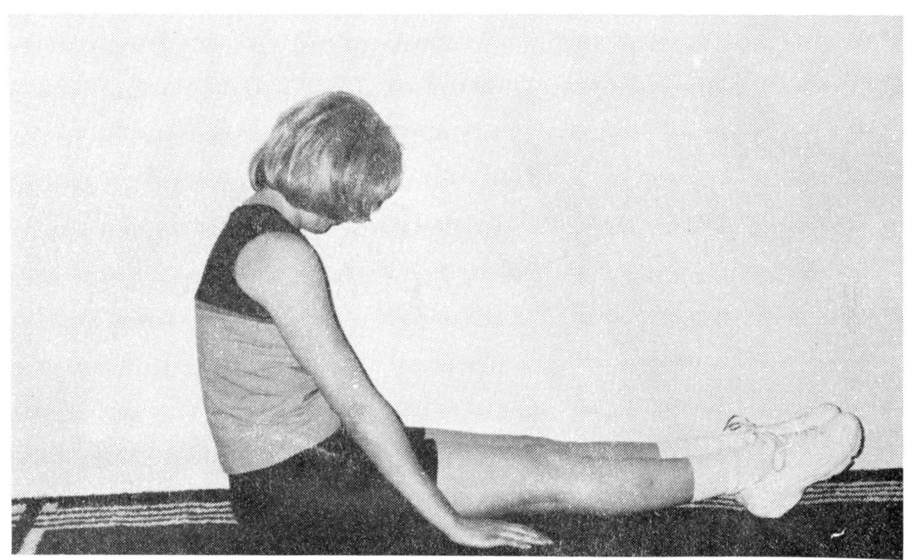

figure 11

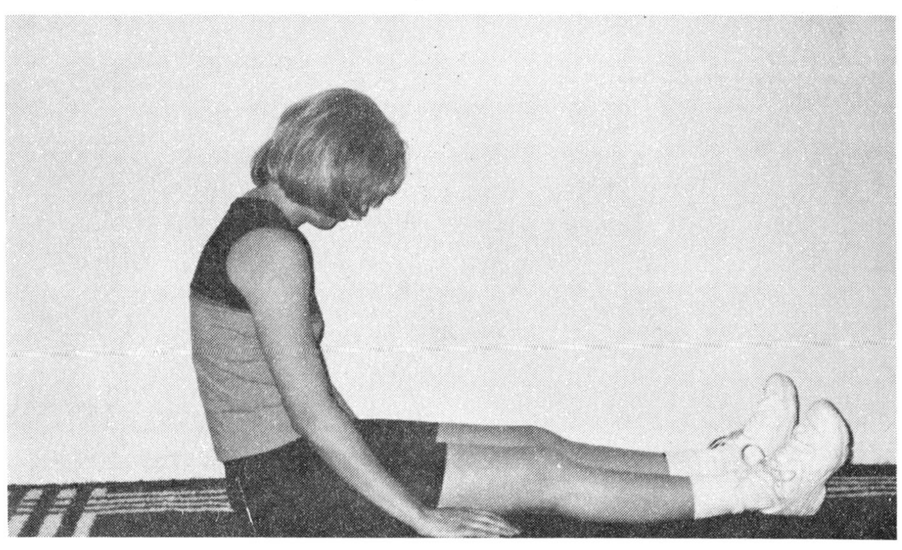

Stand & lunge forward with one leg-don't bend your knee in front of your ankles:

figure 12:

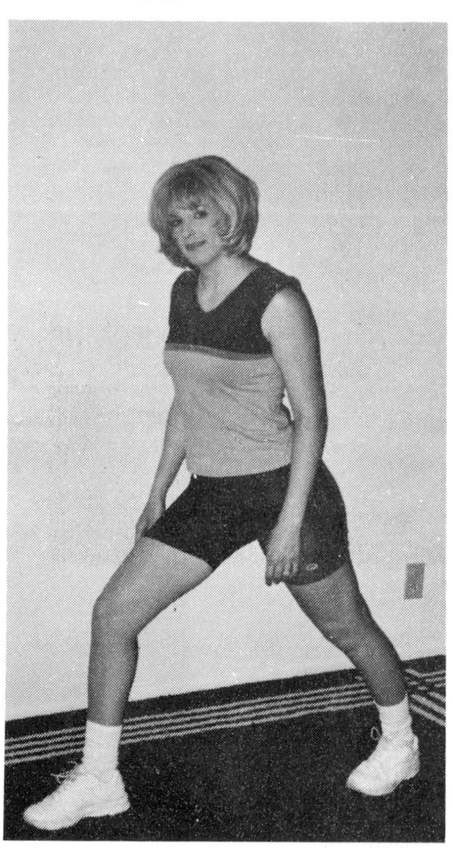

figure 13:

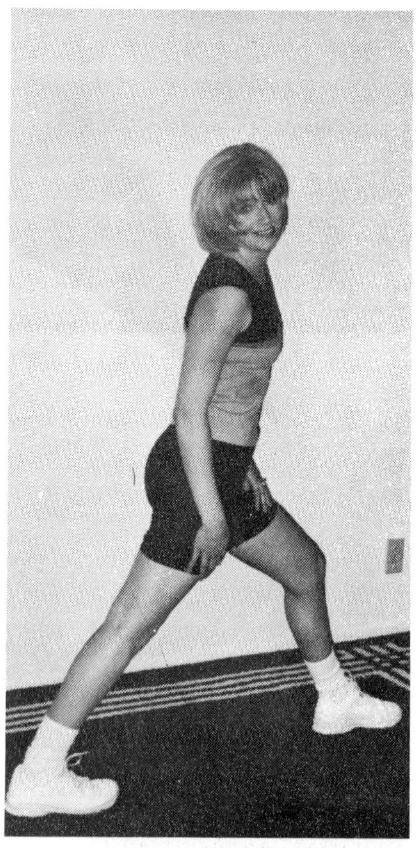

Tense up different parts of your body & then slowly relax them. This example shows the hands.

figure 14:

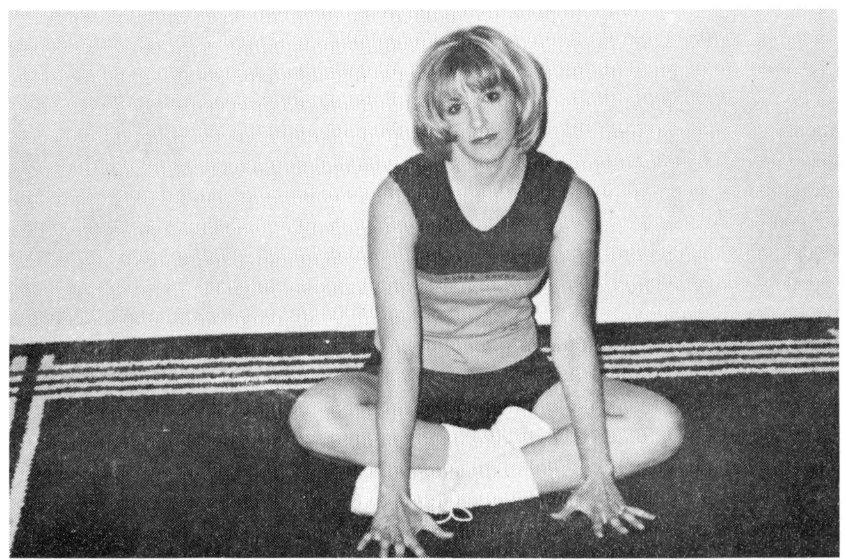

figure 15:

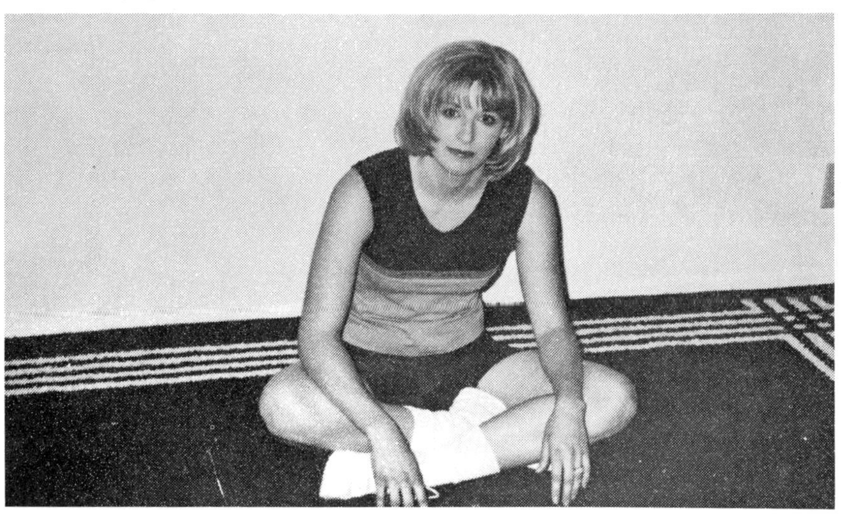

Lie on your back and raise each leg up & down comfortabley. Never do an exercise or stretch if you feel any pain:

figure 16

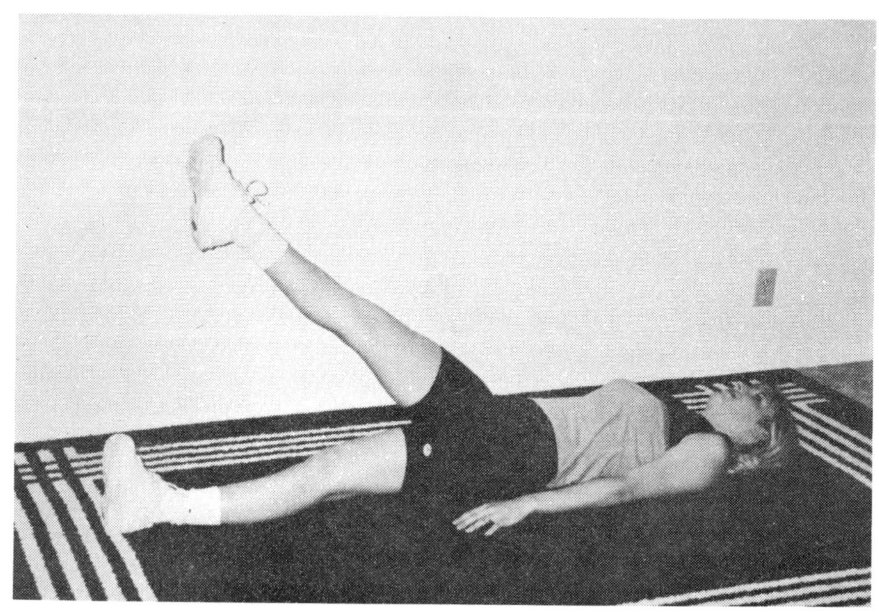

Neck exercises turn neck from left to right, right to left. I find I get more motion if I apply pressure with the stretch!:

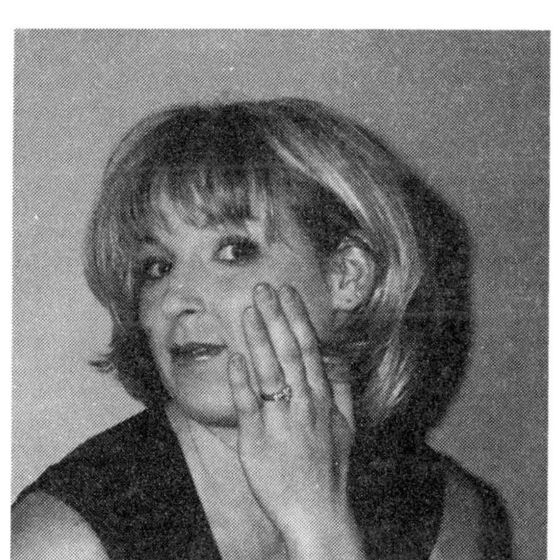

figure 17:

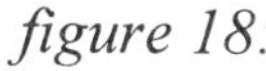

figure 18:

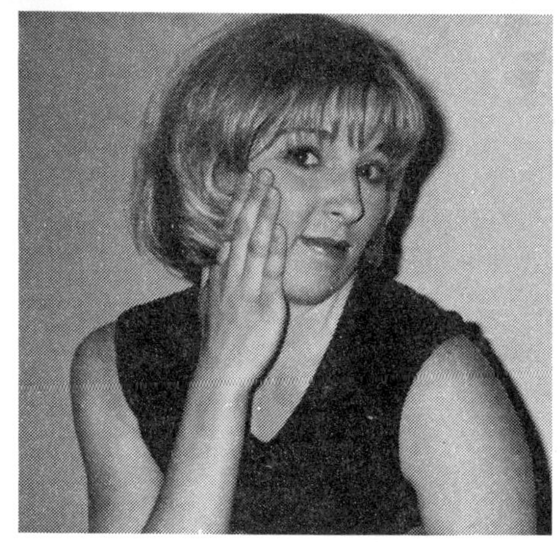

In these neck exercises move your head up and down:

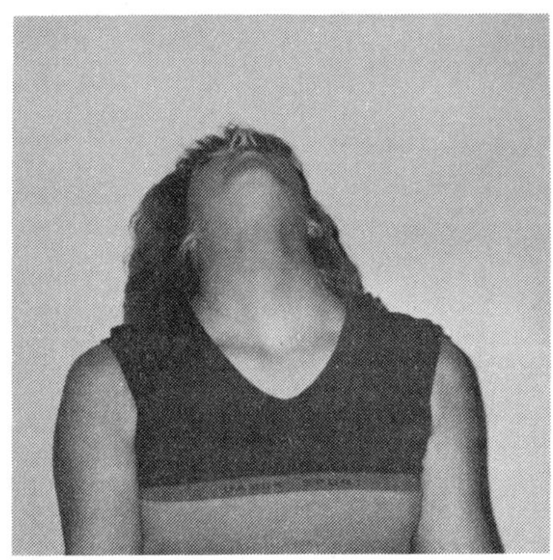

figure 19:

figure 20:

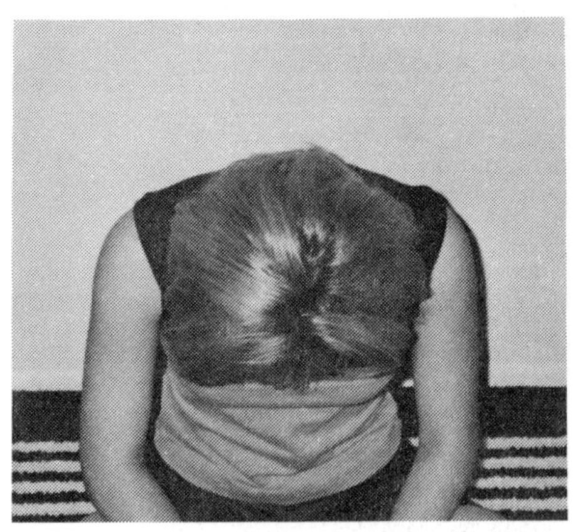

figure 21:

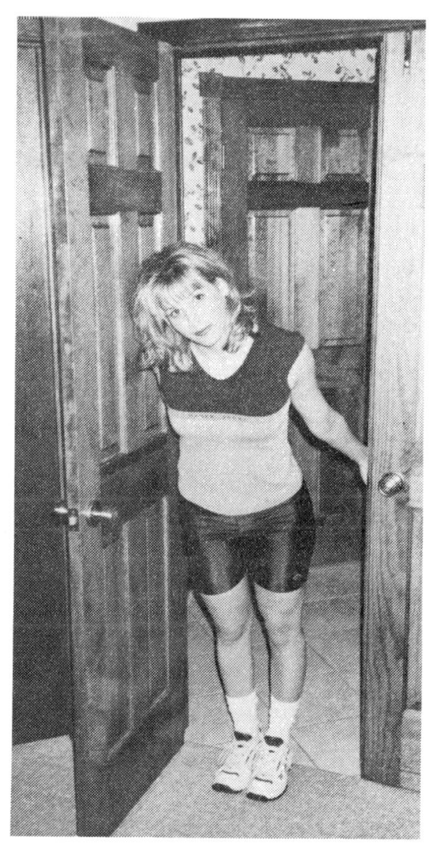

Hold on to the door frame and lean forward!

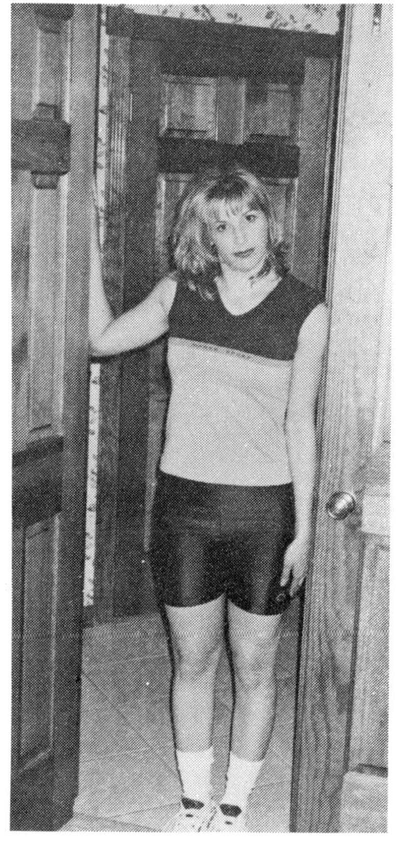

Lean against the doorway and push with the other arm! Do this on both sides !

figure 22:

I found time to stretch even the car ! Reach up and gently press on the inside roof.

(*Do not stretch while driving!*)

figure 23:

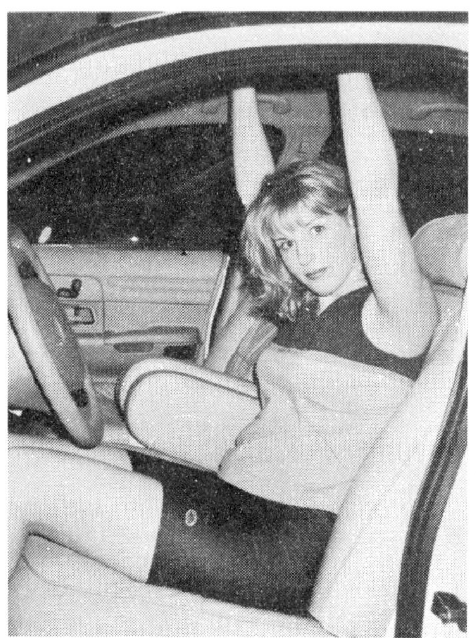

Grasp the steering wheel and push and pull!

figure 24

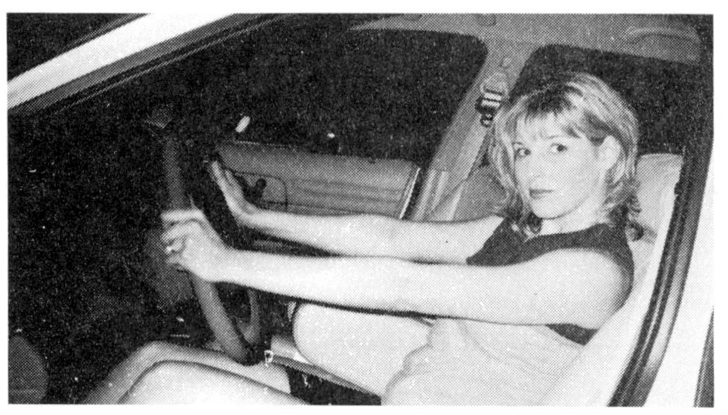

PHYSICAL THERAPY / BODYWORK

Physical therapy involves the use of touch or physical contact of the patient. It incorporates many techniques and methods, but I will limit my discussion to those with which I have had good results, as well as those that have been especially bad for me. Let me affirm that finding the right therapeutic technique can be a great help in controlling pain. The fibromite must explore several to find the best ones for her. Once again, it takes patience and determination.

Physical therapy became useful as a way for me to break the pain cycle, especially during a flare-up. A flare-up would leave me very depressed—I would feel so very incapacitated and so totally hopeless of ever feeling good again. The therapy sessions could ease the pain enough to restore my courage to search again for ways to lift myself out of this debilitating condition.

Several forms of massage are suggested for fibromyalgia syndrome. I've tried several with varying results. Always after a massage, I felt tired, exhausted and usually sore. This, I have since learned, is normal for many people, not just fibromites. However, I found that after a massage, if I went straight home to lie down and rest very quietly for at least thirty minutes, the therapy would have a better effect on my body. During the rest period I would use an ice pack either on the back of the neck or lower back area. I did not always sleep during these rest periods, but the rest itself was helpful. Another important factor to remember with any massage is to drink plenty of water to eliminate toxins. I was surprised by how much more the therapy helped me if I did these things.

My first massage was Swedish massage. It was wonderfully relaxing. However, it failed to reduce the pain I was having. I no longer use this as therapy, although for a wonderful treat I would use it again.

Different doctors suggested different types of massage to try. One recommended accupressure massage. This was a very aggressive and painful therapy that involved deep tissue massage. The massage was so painful that it regularly brought tears to my eyes as it was given. I would then hurt very badly for almost a week; instead of relief, I was in pain constantly and my condition was deteriorating. Again depression overtook me, so I stopped this therapy after a program of two to three treatments a week for several months.

Years before the diagnosis of fibromyalgia, my chiropractor had diagnosed me with myofascial pain, that is pain coming from the fascia (fibrous membrane) of muscles. Years later, when I started massage therapies, I was given myofascial release and craniosacral release massage for the first time. Both of these proved to be beneficial. The myofascial release massage can be a little uncomfortable since the goal is to break up places in the muscle where metabolic wastes have been stored, in other words, to relieve trigger points. The pressure necessary to do this can causes some pain, but not nearly as much pain as the accupressure massage gave me. Since this method of massage involves dislodging toxins, I again drank plenty of water after the sessions to help wash the toxins away—16-24 ounces within an hour after therapy, and more throughout the day. As I said, the massage made me sore, but, unlike the accupressure massage, I would be sore only for that day and maybe the next. I also felt totally exhausted for a while due to the release of toxins. However, after several weeks on the program, the soreness factor improved and I did not feel as weak after the massage sessions.

The craniosacral release massage felt wonderful to me. The purpose was to release tension stored in the connective tissue. I could feel the pain easing away as the massage was being given. The release was significant. I very highly recommend both the myofascial and the craniosacral massage.

Early on, if I missed the massages or did something very physical, I would end up as if I had never started them—back on square one. It was very depressing. To this day, if I experience a flare-up with my TMJ, or any flare-up for that matter, the myofascial and craniosacral release massages are the most beneficial therapy for me. However, though I still use these massages, they are far less frequent and my results last longer since I am on bioidentical hormones.

CHIROPRACTIC CARE

When I was about five years old, I had my first visit to a chiropractor. Dr. Roy Crochet really impressed me because he was so aware of total body health as it related to malfunction anywhere in the body. I am saddened to say that he passed away this year and the many patients he helped will miss him. The main thing that I remember, and a key for my present condition, is the fact that that he did not practice with drugs. He relied more on natural alternatives such as vitamins and herbs. This experience primed me to be willing to try natural remedies even before these became so popular in the US.

According to the American Chiropractic Association and the International Chiropractors Association, it is thought that all bodily functions are controlled by the nervous system. So aches and other maladies may originate from some irritation of nerves from various sources, especially misaligned vertebrae. Chiropractors treat neuromusculoskeletal problems including TMJ and several of the other symptoms I have experienced.

Many of my visits to the chiropractor were to complement the myofascial massage therapy by realigning the vertebrae and the surrounding ligaments. This would help straighten and loosen tight areas so that the myofascial massage was more effective. Muscle tightening can cause subluxations (partial dislocations) of the spine. This can result in severe pain in the neck, shoulder, back, legs, and pelvic area. Sometimes the muscles were so tight that the chiropractor had to use an activator (a small tool used to help patients who tense up and resist the adjustment) to relax me enough to accomplish the adjustment.

Keeping the spine aligned is very important, especially to fibromites. They should continually maintain spinal alignment and use chiropractic and massage as a maintenance program as needed. That way, the body will cooperate with whatever bodywork may be chosen.

BIOIDENTICAL HORMONES

The discussions on hormones in earlier chapters cover much of my history and experiences with hormones. Here, I will discuss the natural hormone program as it was when I started. I will tell how and why I amended it to the program I follow as I write this book. That way, you might benefit from my experiences and find your unique formula faster than I did.

I started using natural hormone therapy in November of 1998. From the start, I used the natural estrogen and the natural progesterone together. I have had to adjust dosages, and it may be that I will have to continuously adjust dosages as my body first achieves and then loses hormone balance throughout my life. However, this constant change may be due to the fact that I take other medications that interfere with hormone absorption. I can deal with that if it continues to help me control the pain of fibromyalgia as it is doing now.

Tri-Est is the name of the estrogen formula I use and it is one of the common bioidentical HRT formulas; it consists of a mixture of 80% estriol, 10% estradial, and 10% estrone. Besides supplementing the estrogens made by the body, the estriol protects against cancer. The cream can be applied alternately to the abdomen and inner thighs or it can be applied vaginally. I apply it every night vaginally. When I started applying the cream vaginally, I was able to reduce the amount of cream and still get the same good results. In fact, I started out on the recommended dose of 1.25 mg. twice a day. At that level, I still had some symptoms of estrogen dominance—stiff, painful joints, severe stiffness in the left side of my neck, migraines, and vaginal dryness. I then reduced the dosage to half of that, and now I am down to half of 1.25 mg. applied only once a day. The decrease from recommended dose may possibly have been needed even if I had applied the cream to the skin sites, and not vaginally.

Additionally, I use a natural progesterone cream every morning. I never use the Tri-Est and the progesterone creams at the same time because doing so caused me to have migraines. My doctor prescribed a 20% cream: I was told to apply ¼ ml. (dollop the size of a large pea) to the inner thigh twice a day for two weeks and then daily, once a day, to the breast area. That proved to be too much; it caused migraines. After a week I got off of the progesterone cream and used only the estrogens. I have now started the progesterone cream again, but I reduced the dose to ¼ of the original dose (¼ large pea size). That is the marvelous thing about the creams—I did not have to toss out a paid-for prescription, I just reduced the amount by any measure I thought proper until the correct amount was found.

After about three months on natural hormone therapy and after adjusting the hormone dosages to my own needs, I was able to reduce my fibromyalgia symptoms by about 90%—maybe more. (Gall bladder medication caused some pain about that time; it was different from the pain of fibromyalgia, and it was listed as a side effect of the medication.) The pain difference has been wonderful. Even my vitamins started working better after my therapy was well on the way.

After well over a year of being on the natural (bioidentical) hormone therapy, my fibromyalgia symptoms are reduced by about 90%—maybe more. I am still following the same regimen of hormone therapy **(Tri-Est and progesterone).** When needed, I incorporate one or more of the other therapies described in the Victory Plan. But this statement makes it necessary to give another explanation—I still have some side effects and pain from the gall bladder surgery I had in February of 1998 and from a fall in November of 1999. I suffered a whiplash aggravating some discs and nerves in my spinal column. Even these setbacks have a positive side, though, because I have been able to rebound from them much, much faster than I would have been able to do before I devised my personal Victory Plan.

Some of the details (see the medical time line for more) of these setbacks demonstrate the effects that medications can have on hormones. First, the gallbladder surgery—one possible side effect of the synthetic hormone therapy (HRT) is diseased gallbladder. The hysterectomy that I could have avoided, had I known about bioidentical hormones earlier, led to synthetic hormone therapy (HRT) that led to gallbladder surgery. The gall bladder surgery caused complications, including digestive problems and severe chronic diarrhea. I took Colestid for its constipating quality for over a year, and finally realized that I had pain, fatigue, and headaches very often about one hour after taking it. I switched to Questran Light; it caused very severe side effects and interfered with my hormones. After four weeks, I stopped the Questran; several other medications were prescribed; none worked. I could not digest food properly and I became dehydrated several times. Also, I lost twenty-five pounds in three weeks; I experienced severe pain; finally, I could not even eat. I quite literally thought I was going to die. **However, during the time I was off of Questran and Colestid, my hormones renormalized—no hot flashes, headaches, or any FMS pain.**

The second setback, an accident, occurred during the Colestid/ Questran ordeal. I fell and suffered a whiplash which caused some damage to my spinal column (discs and pinched nerves). The specialist I went to for the pain caused by the accident gave me cortisone injections. This really upset my hormone balance, which in turn started a flare-up of FMS that lasted about four weeks. I put my Victory Plan back into full force, the physical therapy, magnets, TENS, and more. Now my hormones seem to be back in balance, and the FMS flare-up has subsided. I am still working with the side effects of the Colestid, but they, too, are better.

My condition is better in almost every way on the bioidentical HRT. I have stopped taking all but a few medications. I now sleep very well and wake up feeling refreshed. I have energy that I have not had in many, many years. I can set goals and accomplish them without fear of long, painful setbacks. I only rarely have a migraine unless one is provoked by medication or physical trauma (dental work). Fibromyalgia pain is absent most of the time. My depression is gone—I never dreamed that I would be able to write a book. **I feel like I have a new life.**

CHAPTER FOUR

Medical Timeline

Of

My Life

Originally, the purpose of the medical time line was simply to help in writing the book. However, we decided that the minute details in this time line could possibly help either a patient researcher or a scientific researcher, so we included it in the book. My hope is that it might benefit patients and their doctors; maybe they can draw conclusions from my life that will benefit the treatment of fibromyalgia.

You will notice that I went to many doctors, sometimes several in a week. And it may seem that I sometimes blindly followed bad advice. Well, I did. One explanation for my dedication to following doctors' orders, even when it hurt, was what we were taught as children. The roles in society were clear—doctors played their part and so did we. Our culture taught us that doctors were almost gods. I thought that the doctor could cure anything as long as I was a good patient. By their example, parents taught us not to ask too many questions and that doctors' orders were to be explicitly followed. For years I was very hesitant to question them; it felt disrespectful to do so unless asked. I did finally learn that I absolutely had to ask questions. But only in the last year or so can I say that I feel confident contesting a doctor, and that confidence comes after innumerable, sometimes costly, experiences.

Parental guidance also taught me to consult the doctor before making even the slightest changes in methods or medications; it became my lifelong habit. Added to this habit was the fact that, early on, I was referred to a different doctor for almost every symptom. If my jaw hurt, I went to the oral surgeon for the necessary medication, etc. The doctors seemed to require this. Since they were the experts, and I was learning, I followed this example until quite late in my course of treatment. Only later did I learn that I could have called on the neurologist and my family doctor more. Had I known this, I might have avoided some bad experiences.

The time line is rather complete, but it does not include everything. It does not include my many trips to the chiropractor, for example, since those treatments are mechanical, and not chemical. Depression is usually a significant consequence of fibromyalgia, and the time line does not reflect my total experience with depression. Over the course of the disease, I would become depressed occasionally. Usually this was overcome by the doctor's encouragement or on hearing of a new treatment possibility of any kind. My depression, and anxiety, became severe after the gallbladder surgery when I suffered the life-threatening digestive upset for almost a year. The fact that some of the principle doctors in this ordeal failed to understand how sick I was, caused this acute episode of depression. Moreover, it was a horrible feeling to think that I had conquered the fibromyalgia, and now this side effect of a surgery that should have been avoidable might even kill me.

My contention for years was that hormone imbalance was making me sick. There could be several causes. The allergies I suffered called for cortisone (hormone) shots for a long period. Environmental factors probably played a part, too; it is becoming more accepted that these factors affect hormones. In fact, one particular example of environmental factors may be significant—a man who was later jailed for using illegal and dangerous chemicals sprayed our house for many years. The chemicals were so dangerous that years later, when the danger was learned, families had to move out of their houses for months and have them treated (rather like the asbestos problem). This time line shows some factors and patterns that affected my hormones and contributed to my many fibromyalgia symptoms; we have bolded the ones that are significant in our opinion.

1956. Born May 10, 1956, I was the fourth apparently healthy child of eight children.

1958-1959. I had two childhood incidents. They were medically insignificant, but they did land me in the hospital. One was when I swallowed a drapery hook, which passed through my digestive tract, as the doctor had predicted it would. The other was when I stuck my nose in the crack on the backside of a closet door. My mother closed the door, smashing my nose and lip—that one cured my nosiness.

1961 approximately. I had my first trip to the chiropractor; it was our family habit to visit the chiropractor for almost any illness because he used natural remedies. He found I was not breathing correctly; he compared my breathing to that of a rabbit. In addition to the spinal adjustments he gave, he suggested I do breathing exercises—blowing up balloons.

Even in that early period of my life, I was tired a lot. In fact, I missed many school days (up to sixty in one year) due to fatigue and minor ailments—I had all A's, though, so it was overlooked. I was a "puny" child. I had allergy problems, tonsillitis, and sore throats that lasted into my twenties. I experienced restless nights and nightmares, and I would talk and scream in my sleep about negative things happening. Sometimes I would even sleepwalk. These night activities went on all through my young years. I was very thin growing up. I had tonsillitis quite often. I was taken to the hospital with 105° fever on one occasion; they literally packed me in ice and made me eat ice along with other medical treatments, but I was able to return home on the same day. I was put on vitamins, and because they thought that I was developing rickets, I had to eat sardines for a good while, as well. I got better, but I always was very tired in the mornings.

1964 approximately. I had mumps on one side of my face.

1965 approximately. I had one of the worst cases of chicken pox the doctor had ever seen. I still was having lots of bad dreams as well as sleepwalking and sleeptalking.

1969 approximately. I had a cyst removed from my neck when I was about twelve years old. I had gotten sunburned and the cyst became infected. The cyst had long roots that the doctor had not anticipated, and he cut through an artery while doing the procedure. I bled so profusely that my mother had to leave me there and return with other clothes. While waiting, the nurse had me wrap a sheet around myself and sit in the doctor's private office, bloody hair and all, until my mother returned, because they needed the room for another patient. I was very weak. When I think about that experience, I see just how unprofessionally I was treated. This was my first bad experience in a doctor's office; little did I know that it was the beginning of a journey that would include many more bad experiences.

1969. At 13 years old, the end of 8th grade, I began experiencing migraines before the onset of my menstrual cycles. I had severe heavy bleeding when my cycles did start. I had to leave school on several occasions with severe migraine, severe cramping, and vomiting. I would have to lie in bed and not move to try to cope with the pain, because at that time Tylenol was the only thing available to me. I did not have regular menstrual cycles until after I had my first baby.

1971. At about 15 years, I was playing football with my brother and he accidentally hit my face with the football and broke my glasses and my nose. I did not have surgery and it healed without medical attention. We did not tell my parents.

1972. By about 16 years, I began to ask if I had a hormone problem causing the bad, irregular menstrual experiences because my experience was so different than that of my friends. The doctor said these conditions were normal for some women, and that they would probably self-correct after marriage and giving birth to the first child.

1977, Jan. At the age of 20, I was in a car accident; the chiropractor said I experienced a whiplash. My general practitioner agreed. I experienced daily headaches, migraines, nausea, jaw pain, severe tiredness, and nervousness. I began taking Tylenol daily. I also took muscle relaxants for several months. The insurance company's doctor examined me and, after tests, diagnosed "stress" without a whiplash. I refused the nerve pills they suggested, and began taking Tylenol daily. I continued the chiropractic care for several months, and the pain in my neck subsided. However, the headaches and fatigue worsened after the wreck, and I began having panic attacks.

I was married three months after the wreck on April 9, 1977. Because of what I went through after the wreck, that was a traumatic three months. I was sick with headaches and fatigue for my wedding; I could not even help pick the dresses for the wedding. I was married about a week when I can remember dreaming that we had big spiders in the bed. I was screaming and trying to kill them when my terrified husband woke me up.

1977, May to June. I had a bad bladder infection. I went to the general practitioner who had been our permanent family doctor. **I asked for, and he prescribed, a medication to regulate my periods.**

1977, July. I became pregnant with my first child. **About two months into pregnancy I began to feel much better. I had enormous energy, rare headaches, rare body aches** (until the last heavy month of pregnancy, which is normal), and no jaw pain. I slept well. I even went back to work at very physical jobs—I was a butcher's helper until after my fifth month of pregnancy, and after that, I did house cleaning for many local nurses.

1978, April 3. I was 21 years old. **My first baby was born.** The delivery was normal. I had false labor so realistic that I was admitted to the hospital five times before it was the real thing. On the day of delivery, I went in about six in the morning and had her at three that afternoon.

After we were home for several days, my baby girl had blood in her diaper. The doctor said she had gotten too many hormones from me, and that it would taper off just like a menstrual period does for a woman. I breast-fed her for about six weeks, then I had to stop because my breasts became inflamed.

I became very stressed at being a new mother; this seemed to cause undue tiredness even though I was taking vitamins. I went back to work again. **After about four months, all old symp-**

toms began to ease back, especially migraines, fatigue, and nightmares. I kept working, but I had to reschedule work a lot. I talked in my sleep almost every night.

1981, April. I became **pregnant with my second child,** and this pregnancy was the same as the first. Except for morning sickness that plagued me almost all day for the first few months, **I again felt so much better. I had enormous energy and continued to work until my last week of pregnancy.**

1982, Jan. 21 and 22. I was 25 years old. I started labor pains early one night and had pains all night. At five in the morning they were one minute apart and I decided to go to the hospital. After the five false admittances for my first baby, I intended to be sure before I went in this time. The nurse examined me; she said I was barely dilated and that I should go home. I strongly protested, so she said I could wait a little while if it made me feel better. At 7 A.M. they wanted to discharge me, but I absolutely refused. Before 9 A.M. my water broke; the nurse examined me, and, to her surprise, I was fully dilated. They ran me down the hall, I screamed all the way, and they barely had time to get me on the delivery table before **my baby boy was born on January 22, 1982.** I could not understand why that nurse wanted to send me home, but it is a good thing that I stayed, or I probably would have had my baby in the car. I went home after one night in the hospital.

After one week, my son was choking and not breathing right. The doctor said he had a cold, but when he did not improve, I took him to another doctor. It turned out to be pneumonia and allergies, especially to milk and to penicillin. After two and a half weeks at home, I spent a week in hospital with him; he almost died. I was told that boy babies do not fight for their lives as girl babies do. I had to take him for many injections after we went home and he steadily improved. This was very stressful. The lack of rest kept me from recovering from the delivery. **All my old symptoms came back even while we**

were in the hospital. I had post-partum depression very badly. I would cry for no reason at all.

<u>1982, March and April.</u> About 6 weeks after delivery I finished breast feeding and **started taking birth control pills.** It was one of the stronger ones according to an astonished statement made by another doctor at a much later time.

About this time, I had my first TMJ incident, though at the time I did not know the term (the TMJ diagnosis was not until 1986). During a yawn, my jaw locked open for a few minutes; I had to manipulate it to close it. This started happening more often, and I began to suffer jaw pain at times. I finally went to an oral surgeon. **I asked him if the problem could be from the hormone pills, but he thought that the pill would help, not aggravate, the problem.** He said he did not see anything wrong; he offered nerve pills, which I refused. I treated the symptoms with Tylenol and ice packs.

During the week off the pill, the jaw problems and migraines were worse and occurred more frequently. They became uncontrollable and would not respond to Tylenol during that week. The oral surgeon explained that the migraines worsened around the time of the menstrual cycle because the body swells causing muscle contraction headaches. At the time I accepted this explanation. **I stayed on different forms of birth control for 14 years, but in 1985 my dose was reduced to the weakest one made.**

<u>1983 or 1984</u> I was out of town and experienced the worst migraine ever. I took over-the-counter medicine for pain. I had severe bouts of vomiting all day. Just moving the head would cause me to vomit. I became dehydrated and I didn't know it; I did not even know what dehydration was at the time. Friends insisted that I go to the emergency room. I was in the hospital for three days. The doctor treated me with Demerol for headache. He tested me extensively, including tests for spinal meningitis and diabetes.

My discharge papers said I had diabetes, but when I saw my family practitioner, who again tested for diabetes, he said the test was negative. He explained that the intravenous treatment for dehydration caused a false reading on the diabetes test done in the hospital.

This whole experience was scary because it happened the same week that the news media stated that several people were poisoned with tainted over-the-counter medicine, which I had been using extensively.

1983 or 1984. I had a freak accident when a piece of clothes hanger was shot from under a riding lawn mower and struck me in the temple of my head. I had to go to the emergency room; cat scans showed that the hanger barely missed the optic nerve behind my eye. I bled profusely, but other than being extremely sore, I was not seriously injured, and was released from the hospital.

1985. We moved to Harvey, La. I had my own business repairing windshields, and I also went into a business venture of making cloth dolls. I was the seamstress. That activity was very stressful to my body. I began to suffer severe neck pain, the first since the wreck. **I also continued to suffer with the jaw pain and migraines. It seemed as though if I had neck pain it would induce jaw pain, and if I had jaw pain it would induce neck pain.** I did not realize at the time that this was because there are so many muscles in the neck and the jaw that react to each other.

1986. We moved back to Houma because my father was diagnosed with cancer and we wanted to be near to help with his care and spend quality time with him. I quit my windshield business but continued to make the dolls. I continued to suffer a lot in the neck and shoulders.

I went to Ochsner Clinic in New Orleans where **an oral surgeon diagnosed temporomandibular joint problems (TMJ)**. I saw several other doctors there, as well, because they did a complete physical exam on me. Muscle relaxers, Vicodin as needed for migraines, and Flexeril was the treatment plan. The doctor tried several anti-inflammatory drugs over time, and they all irritated my digestive system. They caused burning in the pit of the stomach and sporadic bouts of diarrhea. I also tried Midrin for migraines. The doctor ordered a mouth splint to be worn all the time to prevent clinching.

I worked with the Ochsner team for over a year; during that time I endured painful tests, treatments, and some dental work. One procedure I remember involved an injection in the jaw joints that allowed the doctors to see the damage in the jaw joints. The chemicals used caused my eyes remain stuck open for several (2-3) hours; I could not blink. That was extremely painful. They also took a MRI of my jaw, and it, too, was painful because of the way you have to bite on a mouthpiece during the procedure.

In spite of all the procedures, the jaw pain worsened, so the doctor ordered jaw surgery. The surgery required that the mouth be wired shut for about six weeks (perhaps months) after surgery. But, because of the former broken nose, I needed to first correct that problem to allow proper breathing while my mouth would be wired shut—a presurgery surgery.

1987, April 1. The nose surgery involved two different procedures. The physician's name was Dr. Butcher, who, by the way, was a warm and caring doctor; the surgery was done on April Fool's Day, but the surgeries went very well. At least it wasn't on Friday the 13th. It is a good thing I am not superstitious.

They put a splint in my nose and told me not to laugh or smile for a week. This is very hard to do if you are told not to do it; I guess it is human nature. Three days after the surgery, three of my sisters were visiting; it was late, and we were watching TV in the dark. The youngest had fallen asleep on the couch. Another sister spilled a very large glass of water in her face; she jumped up in a confused panic with the funniest look on her face. It was one of those "family bumbles" that you remember for years. All of us tried so very hard not to laugh because of my nose splint, but the very act of trying not to laugh made things even funnier. I laughed more than I had in months. I did pay for it in pain the next day.

1987-1988. I continued to get severe **migraines, so bad that I frequently had to seek relief at the emergency room**. Many times I would sit and wait sometimes as much as four to six hours before seeing a doctor there. The shots would be Demerol and something for nausea. I noticed that **each time I got a shot with something for nausea, my body and my bones would hurt;** it felt similar to the way I felt when I was dehydrated. I wondered why this happened.

1988, March. I had temporomandibular joint surgery from 7:00 A.M. to 4:00 P.M. This was the most horrible post-surgical experience I ever awoke to. For one thing, I was totally nude in the recovery room. I was in severe pain and I was alone. No one would come to me in the recovery room, and I couldn't call for help because I had just had jaw surgery. Finally, I noticed a metal object on the bedside table, and I threw it into the center of the room where the nurse's station was. They then came to me; I started hyperventilating and shaking uncontrollably because I was so cold and in so much pain. They put me on oxygen, covered me with warm blankets, and finally gave me something for pain. Why do hospitals allow the staff to treat people this way?

Moreover, I went home after three days in the hospital to suffer unbearable pain. To manage pain, I was told to take one Mepergan (Demerol and Phenergan combined) every four hours and I was given muscle relaxers. It was not nearly enough to stop the pain. Only much later did I find out that I could have taken a double dose for the first week at home.

After several days at home trying to sleep in a recliner, I had to return to the doctor because the pain was unbearable, especially in my ears. My jaw was so swollen that it squeezed my eardrums. The doctor readjusted my splint and allowed me to wear it for the first time since the surgery; that helped to reduce the pain enough that the pain medicine then provided some relief. My face was bruised, discolored, and very swollen. I could not lie down. Each time I would fall asleep, I would be waked up by whole-body jerks. I was miserable. I couldn't chew any food for three months, so I lived on creamy foods, soups, and liquids.

My father passed away during the week after my surgery. The oral surgeon put me on Elavil for a short time, because he was afraid that the stress would cause me to clinch my jaw and suffer a setback in healing from the surgery. The Elavil helped me to sleep better at night, but I did not like the tired feeling I had all day long, so I did not use it very long.

1988. At one of the many surgery follow-up visits, the doctor prescribed more anti-inflammatory medication, Naprosyn. I also had Vicodin and Flexeril as needed for pain and muscle relaxation and TMJ migraines. I took the Naprosyn regularly because it was important to the treatment; the doctor said I would probably need it the rest of my life. I took the Flexeril regularly at first, then tapered off; I avaoided taking the Vicodan until I felt desperate.

The jaw surgery was not successful as far as relieving my symptoms of pain and migraines, but it did allow me to be able to open my mouth wider and it stopped my jaw from dislocating any more.

After the jaw surgery, I began to experience the total body pain for the first time. The oral surgeon worked with me for two more years trying to control my pain.

<u>1989-1990.</u> My neck problems lessened when I quit working on the dolls, but I began to have stomach pains that would not subside. I went to a local internist. The pain was in my upper stomach and right upper side. At first the doctor thought it was ulcers, so he ordered the upper GI series of tests. The results were normal, **so the doctor ordered a gallbladder ultrasound, and it, too, was determined to be normal because I had no gallstones.** The next thing the doctor suspected was a cyst on my pancreas, which really left me panicky because my uncle had died of pancreatic cancer. I had numerous CAT scans done which revealed nothing.

The last tests given were a barium enema and a colonoscopy. The doctor performed this test with me awake and without any pain medication or Valium. I understand that normally something is given for pain because the procedure is so painful. Please do not ever have a colonoscopy without being medicated, because to suffer like this is inhumane, as I was told when I had my next colonoscopy at Ochsners Hospital years later. The results of the tests revealed colon spasms and mucous pockets. I was given Librax. Also, I continued to have the sporadic burning pain and diarrhea which were the side effects of the anti-inflammatory medicines from the TMJ surgery.

During this time I also developed shingles. At first I had a severe ache in my neck for two weeks, and then I developed a small circle of bumps on my neck. This was the same week the movie Arachnophobia came out, and everyone was afraid to tell me they thought a spider had bitten me. I asked the pharmacist and he said it looked like a caterpillar bite. I had not seen the movie, but my best friend and first cousin Mona talked me into going to the doctor. She had seen the movie and just knew that I would have to have my flesh cut out; she did not tell me this, however, until after we went to the doctor. The bumps had gotten pretty large (like chicken pox). The doctor diagnosed shingles and prescribed a topical ointment to use. They cleared up after several months, but I still had the neck and shoulder pain to recur for the next year or two; this is because a nerve is involved.

1990, April 4. The oral surgeon called for an MRI of the jaw because I was still having so much pain. Another jaw surgery was a possibility, but he wanted to try other things first.

1990, April 19. The oral surgeon decided to **refer me to the rheumatology** department at Ochsner Clinic because he thought I **might have a muscle problem he called fibrocitis; he said that many TMJ patients get fibrocitis.** The rheumatologist performed the tender point test. **I later learned that, of the eighteen possible tender points, I reacted to all eighteen points.** I had all-over-body pain, pelvic pain, and burning, stabbing pains—pain so bad that you want to crawl out of your body. (At the time I had access to any medication that I needed, and during a total flare-up, not any of them, or all of them together, could stop the pain.) Other symptoms included restless nights—waking up at night feeling like I was dying; I couldn't breathe. I also had the usual headaches and fatigue. The diagnosis of **fibrocitis was confirmed.**

I was given occupational therapy that included putting my hands in hot wax, squeezing a ball of some type of putty substance in my hands, and learning different stretches to do. I felt more pain because the exercises were too much for me at the time. I was put on muscle relaxers, more anti-inflammatory drugs, and Elavil. The anti-inflammatory drugs (the main one being Relafen) helped with the post-surgical jaw pains. Elavil left me very fatigued, so I tried Pamelor instead. (I worked with this team of doctors for about eight years, and I still sometimes consult them.)

1990-1991. I became legally separated from my husband and had to start working full time, a stressful period. I experienced continued body pain and general headaches for the next several years and continued to suffer from migraines on a monthly basis. I was still on the birth control pill, I had access to pain medications if I needed them, and I continued taking the anti-inflammatory drugs.

I continued my treatments at Ochsners for years—every three months blood tests were done.

1991, November. The **rheumatologist prescribed diuretics;** he thought they would help with the menstrual swelling and resulting headaches. **The diuretics caused severe leg cramps.**

1992, April. A chronic FMS flare-up prompted the **rheumatologist to send me to a neurologist because of severe migraines associated with menstrual periods.** He recommended Flexeril during menstrual periods and continuing the anti-inflammatory medicine; he thought the headaches could be aggravated by caffeine. He is the very wonderful doctor who has treated me since that day. The Anaprox helped the TMJ somewhat, and it helped the headaches a little.

1993, May. The rheumatologist ordered sinus x-rays because of face pain and headaches. Tests proved normal.

1993, November. The ENT doctor who had done the nose surgery, performed a small surgical procedure to make a minor adjustment.

1994, May. I went to an internal doctor because of chest pains, heart palpations, and fast pulse. He diagnosed **mitral valve prolapse** and gave me Inderal. The condition continued to affect me every few months until I started using the bioidentical hormones.

1994, August. I had a colonoscopy at Ochsner Clinic because I had some stomach problems from taking the anti-inflammatory medications. Since I had not had one in about five years, and since colon cancer has afflicted my immediate family, my rheumatologist felt that it was needed. The results were normal. (My Father died in 1988 as a result of colon cancer and my sister had surgery approximately three years later for cancer of the colon. (In 1998, my brother was diagnosed with colon cancer. Early detection spared his life. I cannot emphasize how important it is to do regular screening for cancer!!!!)

1994, October. At Ochsner Clinic, the oral surgeon called for another MRI on the jaw. This latest MRI revealed that I needed another jaw surgery, but the doctor recommended that we not do it because he could not be sure of the results—there was a greater chance that I would be in more pain after surgery with less chance for improvement. So, the doctor started me on a series **of cortisone and Healon injections in the jaw joint.** The first series of three helped the jaw pain significantly but simultaneously caused a flare-up of FMS. The second series was helpful, too. **But the third series (starting August, 1995) left the right jaw joint in excruciating pain, and I still have intermittent pain in that joint today.** That was the end of those treatments, and that was my final answer.

I also was regularly seeing the orthodontist who had treated me even before the TMJ surgery. He was mainly trying to keep my teeth and jaw in proper alignment, a necessity for TMJ patients. I continued to wear the splint constantly and I still use a splint today.

Also, **I was still getting the migraines and going to the emergency room** too often. On my last trip there for a migraine, I waited four hours to see the doctor; I was vomiting and afraid that I would dehydrate again. I was in terrible pain, and the only thing they gave me was a remedy for nausea. I did not realize this until I went home and suffered from the migraine for the entire night. The next morning, I called to see what pain medicine I had received as it had not worked, and that's when I found out that I had received only nausea medication.

After that very painful episode, my oral surgeon prescribed Imitrex injections for the migraines. I could give them to myself at home. The injections worked very well. I also tried the pills, but the results were not as good. I used the Imitrex rather often, up to twice a month, until I got on bioidentical hormones. I was glad when I no longer needed the Imitrex because of the side effects. After being on it for a while, I began to suffer from tightness in the throat, racing heartbeat, and dizziness. At one time, I tried another similar medication. It caused chest pains, too, so I now use Midrin for migranes from the disk problem in my neck. But, the Imitrex is so effective for migraine headache that I have used it again once or twice, despite the side effects, instead of going to the emergency room.

1994, November. I fell down my stairs and landed on the third to last step with one leg up and one leg down. The fall caused an extreme flare-up of fibromyalgia, and caused leg pain and lower back pain. I went to a chiropractor for months and worked with the physical therapist there. The therapist noticed knots all over my body, but they were expecially large in the thigh area; he remarked that I had more trigger points than most patients. This was my first accupressure therapy, and it was extremely painful for me.

The physical therapy was not really helping, and my husband encouraged me to rule out back injury, so I went to an orthopedic doctor for lower back pain. But he just looked at the chiropractor's x-rays, did a brief exam, and said to continue the physical therapy if I wanted to. He was in and out so fast; he was not interested. I have had these disappointing appointments before—in so much pain and it seems as though the doctor does not even try to solve the problem.

I went back to my rheumatologist. He gave me two cortisone injections in the lower back; it did help the lower back pain, but none of the other symptoms, and my FMS flare-up remained.

1994, December. I remarried and my husband has been very loving and supportive through this whole ordeal. It is very important to have someone to talk to about your pain and your disappointments, as well as your victories, when you are fighting such a battle. Also, I had the second series of jaw injections (cortisone and Healon) mentioned above.

1995, May. I was still trying to resolve the migraines and I knew hormones were the cause. I went to a gynecologist and told him my theory. He told me to take Premarin for a few days before and after my period to help boost the estrogen. I was to continue

the regular use of the birth control pill that I was already on. It did not work, so he prescribed a different birth control pill that I was to take non-stop, with no breaks at all. I got a second opinion, and decided not to do it. I was afraid of it.

1995, August. I had the third, and last, series (mentioned above) of cortisone injections in the jaw. At that point, I was discouraged with the treatments.

1996, July 31. I consulted with an endocrinologist because I was convinced that the migraines were hormone related. (The muscle contraction headaches from TMJ had improved from taking the anti-inflammatory drugs, the pain medication, and the Elavil.) **Although I had suffered from migraine headaches since I began to menstruate, after the second baby they became somewhat regular—they were much worse and more frequent during the week that I was "off" the birth control pill.**

When I phoned for the appointment, I made a point to ask if this doctor specialized in hormones and headaches, and I was assured that he did. I had so many medical expenses that I wanted to avoid more appointments where you find out that the doctor cannot help you only after the high fees are paid. I felt like I was going in circles—pay money, no help.

The doctor called for many blood tests to check for several different things (diabetes, hormone levels, cholesterol levels, etc.) Coincidentally, the very next day I had a migraine headache, so I called his office and asked for Imitrex (since that had helped the migraines before). I was told that he did not treat migraines and that I would have to call whoever had previously prescribed it before. What is wrong with this picture—is it just a money thing to some doctors? I went there to be treated for migraines and he wouldn't prescribe anything for me. Imitrex is not an addictive drug or a narcotic. I had asked about headache treatments before going there; I had just spent over three hundred dollars in consultation and blood test fees; now, the very next day it was as if I had never been there and he would not give me the medicine I needed. Thank God for my gynecologist. I called him and he immediately called in a prescription for Imitrex for me.

1996. I saw a documentary on TV about endometriosis and this seemed to describe my leg pain. So off I went to the gynecologist. He suggested a laparoscopy (an endoscope that allows visual examination of the abdominal cavity). My insurance plan entered the picture, though, because my coverage would pay 80% for a "plan" doctor, instead of 60% or 40% for doctors not on the list. Due to the expense involved, I did choose a plan doctor, and he scheduled a laparoscopy and hysteroscopy (exploring the uterus with a special endoscope through a small incision).

The results were more than I expected—endometriosis, a fibroid tumor on the uterus, and a prolapsed uterus. The doctor performed a D&C procedure. I had not had a problem with heavy bleeding since I had been on the birth control pills, but after this procedure, I bled so much that I thought I was hemorrhaging. The bleeding continued for four or five days.

Even worse, I had a bad reaction to the anesthesia used in the operating room. They had started an I.V., and as we were talking, a sudden, very hot feeling began to come over me from my head down to my waist; I felt weak, like I was going to die. I tried to tell them, but my body was paralyzed and I couldn't speak. This lasted about a minute and then I fell asleep. I found out later that there were two chemicals used that usually are mixed together ahead of time. But this time, they gave me one before the other, and that is why I fell asleep after not being able to move. This really traumatized me, so now I ask extensive questions about any procedure that will be done to me and what possibly could go wrong.

1996. After the laparoscopy, I had a problem with my jaw being swollen and painful from being manipulated during surgery. I also had trouble and pain swallowing because the tube they put down my throat injured the uvula—because of my TMJ condition, they just barely opened my mouth and forced the breathing tube down my throat. (For my next surgery, I made sure they opened my mouth correctly.) My surgery was on a Wednesday; by Friday I had to see a doctor for my throat.

My throat was in bad shape. I phoned around and found a throat specialist who was the only one with an opening in his appointment book and who was able to take me pretty much anytime that day. (A bad sign—if a specialist has a lot of openings, you'd better check him out). Then began a series of very, very strange events. First, I was in the waiting room and my chair collapsed. No one came to see about me— no nurse, no receptionist, nor anyone. I was already in pain before I got there, and then I had this fall! The fall was upsetting—all I wanted to do was see the doctor and then go back home to bed. My mother asked for some water so I could take some pain medicine. The office assistants took forever and acted like it was too much trouble to help us.

Finally, I was called to the back to be examined. The doctor that came in was very jolly. First of all, he told me about names—my name, my mom's name—and that his wife was pregnant and he was looking for names for his baby. I told him I was in extreme pain and asked that he just examine my throat quickly so I could go back home and lie down. The chair I was sitting in now had a very high, adjustable back, and the doctor decided he wanted to remove the back so I would be more comfortable. He started fumbling with it and almost knocked me in the head; it made me nervous after just having fallen in the waiting room. He kept fumbling with the chair, and I kept insisting that it was just fine as it was. Right then, the chair came apart, almost sending him flying across the room.

Next, he wanted to show me a picture album of his wife. Again I told him to please just examine me, that I did not feel well enough to look at pictures. He still insisted, and went out of the room to get the album. While he was out of the room, I asked my mom if she thought we might be on the *Candid-Camera* show because this was such an unreal experience. The doctor came back, and finally, after showing his pictures, he examined my throat.

Then, the clincher of this horrible doctor's visit, he informed me that, because of the fall in his office, he was going to examine the incisions from the hysteroscopy and laparoscopy. I absolutely refused because the bandage had not yet been removed by the gynecologist. I pointed out that he was a throat specialist and not a gynecologist, and I told him that I did not feel comfortable with him examining the hysteroscopy site because that is a very discreet area. He kept insisting, so I told him that my gynecologist was nearby and that I would go there. He insisted on calling the gynecologist before I could leave; I felt like a prisoner. I went straight to my gynecologist. Since then, others have told me about strange and hilarious visits with that doctor. The treatment he gave me was an over-the-counter saline spray.

1996. The result of the laparoscopy and the hysteroscopy was that my gynecologist suggested a choice of either a partial or a full hysterectomy to solve my several symptoms. Since I had stopped the anti-inflammatory medicine, my jaw was in extreme pain after the procedures, as well as from the fall in the throat doctor's office. The Tylenol #3 I was taking was not doing anything for my pain.

1996. I decided to get a second opinion at a fertility institute. I was told that they specialized in endometriosis. **The doctor there recommended that I try a series of injections (hormonal) to try to put the endometrioses in remission and avoid surgery. I did try several of these injections, but they left me in worse pain than before, so I stopped the treatments. This failure caused us to**

elect the full hysterectomy because I was assured that it would prevent the endometriosis from returning. The doctor explained that he could just fix the uterus, but that the endometriosis often comes back if both ovaries are not removed.

The thought of a hysterectomy was very hard for me because I did want one more child. I decided to get one more opinion from another specialist in endometriosis. His opinion was to just remove the endometriosis, fix the uterus, and leave one or both of my ovaries.

All three doctors agreed that the endometriosis was more likely to return if the ovaries were left in. I decided on the full hysterectomy. **It seemed so easy to have the full hysterectomy and then get on hormone replacement therapy (HRT).** I thought this was the only way the endometriosis would not return. Little did I know that the endometriosis could return anyway, and that HRT could cause just as much pain as I was already in. We then scheduled the surgery; I thought I was on my way to better health—false hopes again.

1996. Before I had the hysterectomy, I saw an orthopedic surgeon for pain in my neck, back, and legs. I wondered if there might be some damage from the fall in the throat doctor's office, but I knew some of the pain was from the fibromyalgia and the endometriosis. **He gave me several cortisone injections in the neck to ease tight knots.** Also an MRI showed that I had three bulging disks, which many people have, but mine were not bulging in a way to need surgery. The MRI of my back was normal. His opinion was that no damage resulted from the fall.

1996. Also before the hysterectomy, the gynecologist who was to perform the surgery suggested that I have a biopsy of the large knots in my legs. He did not think that they were endometriosis, which I had suggested after reading that endometriosis can occur anywhere in the body, but he admittedly could not explain them either. The biopsy showed the knots to be benign.

1996. In late October and early November I had a recurrence of shingles in the same area on my neck as before. I went to an internal medicine specialist who treated me with Zovirax, topically and also orally (oral could maybe prevent recurrance). The first time I had shingles, they treated me with topical ointment only, and they came back. Also, my gynecologist rescheduled my hysterectomy for a few weeks later because of the shingles. He said that some hormonal injections to be used after surgery could cause the shingles to flare up.

1996, December 19. I almost cancelled my surgery because of an incident with the specialist who was to do the hysterectomy. I should have cancelled, but I did not do it because he was on my insurance plan.

My oral surgeon and my rheumatologist were willing to talk to the specialist to explain how my jaw and my body would react to the trauma of surgery. I, too, explained that I would probably have a severe FMS flare-up after surgery. I told him that I had suffered so much in the past that I wanted to prevent this acute and chronic pain as much as possible. He said he did not need to talk to my doctors; that he well understood my conditions; and that he would not let me suffer needlessly. I felt let down—I knew he really did not under stand this chronic pain, and I knew that the other two doctors would really explain my situation in detail.

I had chosen this particular doctor (from the PPO list) because I thought that an endometrial specialist would give me superior care and treatment, and would be better for my particular symptoms. I went to the hospital to pre-admit, and the feeling of being locked into a bad situation overwhelmed me; I began to cry. This doctor was cold and incompassionate; it showed in the way he talked to me. I was convinced that I needed this surgery so I could get well. I went ahead with it, hoping for the best.

The night before my hysterectomy I had to drink a gallon of liquid to cleanse the colon. After consuming half the liquid, I began to vomit. I called the pharmacist and he said to wait one hour and try again. I tried again and continued vomiting and having diarrhea. I ended up with a migraine headache. I had to take an Imitrex injection. By morning, the headache was gone, but the usual weakness that is an after effect of a migraine was still with me.

I arrived at the hospital early the next day and the surgery was performed as scheduled. After surgery, I woke up in extreme pain and was given a morphine injection. The doctor did not order an intravenous drip for pain medication as most doctors do. I had to wait each time for four hours for pain injections, and even then the nurses were slow to provide them. I was in extreme pain. Each pain injection had to be followed by an injection for nausea, and by the time Friday came, I was extremely sore at the injection sites. The doctor stated that he could not understand why I was in so much pain; he was clueless and totally without compassion. He had just taken out my ovaries, my uterus, and removed endometriosis from my other organs and he couldn't understand how painful this was. I felt like suggesting that we castrate him and see how it felt in two days.

The doctor discharged me with twelve Vicodin tablets. I asked for Lorcet instead, because I tolerated it better, but he insisted that they were the same. I came home and took one Vicodin and vomited and started having bouts of diarrhea. I went from Friday night to Monday morning fighting diarrhea and could not take anything for pain. I called Saturday for Lorcet and he phoned it in to the pharmacy, but I could not hold down any medicine by that time.

Early Monday morning, I called requesting an office visit because I was so sick and still had the diarrhea. The nurse put me on hold; she then came back and told me that the doctor said that, if I still felt the same way tomorrow, to call then for an appointment. I exploded with anger because I knew that my first instinct about him had been correct. I told her to forget it and that I would go to our local emergency room. After the ordeal was over, my husband reported the doctor to our insurance company with the comment that such a man should not treat even our animals. I never saw that doctor again.

I went to the emergency room and waited six hours before I was admitted to the hospital; I was there for a week. My heart rate was over 150 and I had dehydrated. I was admitted with a morphine I.V. pump. They stopped my diarrhea, and put me on intravenous fluids for three days. They did tests on my colon in the hospital; I had to drink a liquid for the tests, and it caused incessant diarrhea. That was at 7 P.M., and by 9 P.M I knew I would dehydrate again if they did not do something. They had taken me off of the I.V. fluids. I requested Kaopectate. The nurse did not want to give it to me because she could not do so without first checking with the doctor on call. She did not want to call the doctor on call (he was taking my doctor's calls) because she was scared to call him after 9 P.M. My husband demanded that something be done. She called him, and then told us that he had "jumped all over her" for calling so late about someone with diarrhea. I received a small amount of Kaopectate that night. The next day when I asked the doctor about "last night," he apologized for what happened; he then called a gastroenterologist in to see me because they could not find the cause of the diarrhea.

According to the gastroenterologist, the specialist had used too many antibiotics in my hysterectomy, and these caused major problems in my colon. I had to give stool specimens and begin a regimen of stomach care. They put me back on intravenous morphine because I had such painful spasms in the stomach and in my back. I had to be treated with an intravenous flow of Flagyl. I was given Bacid to put the good bacteria back in the colon, Diflucan because I now had a yeast problem, Levbid for colon spasms, and Zantac. Can you imagine the pain of having a complete hysterectomy followed immediately by a whole week of incessant diarrhea? Still today I cannot take very much antibiotic medication without suffering intestinal problems. I always use acidophilus before, during, and after I take antibiotics, and it helps.

The whole horrible ordeal was so unfair and so avoidable—especially at the hands of a doctor who assured me of his grasp on my unique problems, and who refused the counsel of my other specialists. The good thing to come from this horrible experience was that a wonderful local gynecologist I had previously seen took over my case. I stayed on the Levbid and the Zantac after going home, and the regimen was beginning to help my digestive problems.

<u>1997.</u> When I finally went home from the hospital, I was in extreme pain—from a flare-up of FMS and TMJ, from back pain caused by colon spasms, and from surgical pains. The gynecologist did not want to give me pain medication because he thought the gastroenterologist should do it. After several phone calls, the gastroenterologist called in a prescription and gave me a stern warning that he would not get me any more.

Few doctors wanted to prescribe pain medication at the time, especially for me who had fibromyalgia, a condition that they considered invalid. Maybe it was that doctors were "under the gun" at the time for overprescribing narcotics, or because they thought FMS could be treated satisfactorily with anti-inflammatory drugs. Whatever the reason, I was hurting; I had never abused narcotics, in fact, I avoided them as much as possible. But, I had just had serious surgery causing serious flare-ups, and no doctor wanted to address my needs. Such treatment made me feel ashamed—I perceived that they thought I was begging for narcotics.

Still in pain, I went to the general practitioner who knew my situation. He told me about a very good fibromyalgia specialist in New Orleans, a rheumatologist (not an Ochsner doctor) who supposedly had the best and latest treatments. I went to the specialist hoping that he might have something new. I explained how badly I was suffering. He ordered blood tests to rule out other diseases that mimic FMS, the same tests I'd had so many, many times. I told him that the anti-inflammatory medicine helped my jaw pain, but if I took two in a day, it would cause diarrhea. If I reduced the dose to one a day, it failed to affect the jaw pain. Neither did it help the fibromyalgia pain. Despite my input, he prescribed a stronger preparation of the same medication, Relafen, one a day, along with Elavil. He, too, refused me any pain medication.

I broke into tears in his office because three supposedly intelligent doctors—a gynecologist, a rheumatologist, and a gastroenterologist—were treating me and none of them would address my pain. They just let me suffer. I was in a bad situation; I was suffering with severe pain and digestive problems, and all they wanted to do was nothing.

1997, March-May. I phoned the oral surgeon (Ochsner) who phoned in pain medication for me several times until I could see the neurologist again.

1997. I saw the gastroenterologist, the one from the local emergency room, several times for about three months; and then when (several months later) it was time to refill my prescription for colon spasms (Levbid), the nurse said they would not refill it unless I had a colonoscopy. This would have been fine except that I had one pill left, and I needed some until she could schedule it. At first she even said that they had never put me on Levbid, but I had the bottle with the doctor's name on it. She was very rude, but I persisted, so she finally found the record showing that they had indeed prescribed it. The nurse's refusal to refill the prescription left me with the prospect of daily bouts of diarrhea. That was very unreasonable of her, and somewhat dangerous for me. I decided to go back to Ochsner Clinic where my care had been consistently good.

1997, June. I went back to the Ochsner neurologist—my longtime home base. **His answer to my problem with the post-hysterectomy hormone injections was to get a gynecologist to prescribe**

smaller doses of hormones to be taken daily. He also suggested that I use the Imitrex, the anti-inflammatories, Elavil, Xanax, and pain medication if needed. He gave me a B12 injection and a prescription; he wanted me to do physical therapy. He recommended a fibromyalgia book to me, the Starlanyl and Copeland book, *Fibtomyalgia & Chronic Myofascial Pain Syndrome: A Survival Manual.*

1997, July. I made another follow-up trip to the neurologist with the same migraines, and now colon problems, as well.

1997, September. In the meantime, I called my family practitioner, and he called in Levbid until Ochsners could see me—almost a month later. I saw a gastroenterologist who ordered another colonoscopy, the third. Just as before, there were no problems with my colon except spasms of the colon. I started questioning; if nothing was wrong, why so many severe problems? **I began to connect the digestive problems to the hormone injections after the hysterectomy.**

1997, November. I went for another scheduled visit to the neurologist. The same symptoms persisted—FMS, TMJ, mitral valve prolapse, and migraines. **But I was now having a few good days (I had started using magnets)**; I was less depressed using the Xanax; and the book and the massage therapy seemed to be helping some.

1997. The post-hysterectomy hormone injections failed to help the pain, headaches (not migraine), and loss of libido, but they did stop the hot flashes and vaginal dryness. After three weeks, the effects of the injection would wear off, and I would get hot flashes and migraine headaches, along with the other symptoms. I next tried the hormone patches (Climara). They mitigated the fibromyalgia pain better, but again, the dose would not last the intended seven days, and I would suffer the effects of unbalanced hormones. I would have a few good days followed by many bad days. By January of 1998, I started vomiting and having pain in my right side, along with some diarrhea; I often thought it was food poisoning, but **I was starting to have gallbladder attacks.**

1998, January. I went to see my internal specialist. He ordered two gallbladder tests; **they showed a diseased gallbladder, but without stones. This disease resulted from the hormone replacement therapy, I am sure. I say this because the laparoscopy in 1996, about three months before the hysterectomy, had shown no disease in any organs, including the gall bladder, except for the endometriosis. Also, one of the side effects listed in the literature for HRT is possible diseased gallbladder. The doctor said I needed gallbladder surgery.**

1998, February. I had gallbladder surgery. After the surgery, I started having chronic diarrhea. I was put on a medication called Colestid for its constipating effects; this did stop the diarrhea, but after a while on it, I began having leg pains (different from the FMS pains) after taking the pill.

1998, March. I had switched back to hormone injections due to the new digestive problems. But, because I had to go in every three weeks, the doctor and I decided to try the Estrace (2 mg.) pills. They did not agree with me at all, and besides, they were less effective than the injecions for hot flashes and some of the other symptoms. The doctor thought I was not absorbing the Estrace, so I tried the patch again for a couple of months.

1998, June. None of the hormone treatments were working, so I went to the doctor who had given me the second opinion before the hysterectomy. Maybe he could offer something new. Besides, it was time for a total gyncecological check up and a mammogram. I went in with the new suspicion of a connection between the hormones and my pain. He ordered a pituitary gland MRI, which showed a normal gland. **Since I complained of loss of libido, along with the severe pain and migraines, the doctor gave me an injection of estrogen and testosterone. The shot did not help any of the symptoms, and I felt worse; I called the doctor about a week after the shot. He prescribed a testosterone pill, Halotestin, 10 mg tablets,**

on July 7, 1998. The Halotestin gave me immediate migraines that nothing could relieve. I had to wait for the effects of the shot and the Halotestin to wear off.

After a month, the doctor gave me a double dose of the hormone shot—10 mg. instead of the usual 5 mg. He thought that perhaps I needed more hormones. That shot caused the worst FMS flare-up I had ever had. It lasted until the effects of the shot wore off. Also, the fact that I had started having pelvic pain again made the doctor think that my endometriosis had returned. He suggested another laparoscopy. I could not believe this; removal of the ovaries was supposed to have prevented the return of endometriosis.

I now had proof—when the effects of the hormone shot wore off, my fibromyalgia pain abated. I knew that the hormones were causing my horror-moans. I decided not to go back to this doctor for more treatment.

1998, June 24. I received a letter from **Tulane University Medical Center** inviting me to participate in a fibromyalgia study in collaboration with the **Ochsner Rheumatology Clinic**. The study had as a premise that environmental factors may play a role in the cause fibromyalgia. I did participate; in August I gave blood for the study; **at that time I shared my opinion that hormone therapy was causing my FMS flare-ups.**

1998, August. I started my own research on hormones (not FMS); my first book was *Smart Medicine for Menopause*, by Sandra Cabot, M.D. The book tells about natural alternatives to synthetic hormones; it confirmed what I had learned from experience. About the same time, a chiropractor showed me a video on the same topic; it was Dr. John Lee (*What Your Doctor May Not Tell...)* discussing his experiences with patients and bioidentical progesterone cream. I saw a Julian Whitaker, M.D., book discussing these same topics. I went to the health food store where the sales person (the sales staff in such stores often know a lot) suggested progesterone cream and gave me a pamphlet on integrative medicine. **I went back to using the hormone patch Climara once a week, along with the progesterone cream for about two weeks, until I could get an appointment with an integrative medical doctor.**

<u>**1998, September.**</u> The integrative medical doctor gave me a physical exam and extensive blood tests. She decided to try different hormones along with other vitamins and supplements. I was given an intravenous mixture (Meyer's cocktail) of vitamins and minerals to try to help build up my immune system. **She told me to continue using the hormone patch and the progesterone cream. She also prescribed Thyroid, 15mg., because of low morning temperature, even though the blood test showed normal thyroid function. This combination did not help me, so the doctor thought I should try Estratest (estrogen and testosterone pill). This aggravated the fibromyalgia pain and headaches. Moreover, I had terrible hot flashes. She stopped the thyroid medication and prescribed the natural (bioidentical) hormone creams that I had just read about. It was the Tri-Est estrogen, 1.25 mg. twice a day, and bioidentical progesterone, 10 PLO once a day.**

The prescription came by mail from Birmingham, Alabama. **However the hormones were mixed in a cream, and it was too strong for me; I had the same reaction as from the too-strong injection.** The doctor had prescribed the hormones separately so that I could adjust dosages, so they refilled my prescription correctly. **I was able to use less then, but I still had some hormonal migraines. However, a lot of my FMS symptoms were much better within two weeks.**

Just as I was starting to feel better, the doctor moved out of state. That meant I had to find another doctor locally who would use natural hormones. **Also, since I was still having migraines and other**

symptoms, I thought that the hormones were not working, or, more likely, I was not using them correctly; whatever the case, I needed some further guidance from a doctor. Since my doctor was no longer there, I looked for another doctor who would help me continue this program.

1998, October. **In a scheduled visit to the neurologist, I told him I had changed hormones and that I was doing better. I told him again that I thought that all along my problem had been hormone-related. He referred me to an endocrinologist who specialized in hormones.** (My appointment was for November.) **He recommeded the book *Screaming to be Heard, Hormonal Connectons Women Suspect...and Doctors Ignore* by Elizabeth Vliet, M.D.**

1998, October 24. I saw another doctor whose receptionist **had assured me by phone that she prescribed "natural" hormones.** I was hoping for help to continue adjusting the Tri-Est and the bioidentical progesterone. I went in with a list of questions; the doctor was in and out of that room in a flash; **the nurse came back in with the prescription already written.** I objected and mentioned that I still had questions. The doctor came back only very briefly. **She convinced me that what I needed was Premarin; she said that it *was* natural;** we would start with that; I should stop using the creams I had. She told me that the creams were not easily absorbed, and therefore, the amount of hormone delivered to the system was uncertain. She trusted the Premarin to deliver a specified amount of hormone to the body. She left again without giving me a chance to ask any more questions. I told the nurse I had more questions; she went out, then came back in, and informed me in a rude manner that if I had more questions, I would have to make another appointment. Such treatment when my insurance plan fully covered this visit!

The doctor's arguments overwhelmed my resolve for several reasons. The **creams had not worked perfectly, though I later found**

out that I had not given them enough time. The doctor had said that Premarin was natural, and although I was uncertain, maybe she was right; after all, the concept of natural hormones was very new to me, so I doubted my own knowledge. There were discussions in the news questioning "natural" remedies, even news of deaths from such remedies.

I followed her guidance with reservations. **I found out weeks later, when I was in severe pain, that these were not the natural-to-the-body, bioidentical hormones. It clinched my feeling that I needed the bioidentical hormones, even though I had not gotten perfect results from them. I felt so close and yet so far—where would I find another doctor to help in this way?**

<u>1998, October.</u> **At least three times, I had chest pain attacks that would radiate up through the throat and into the jaw.** The cardiologist ordered an ultrasound; it showed an 80% blockage in the carotid artery. He performed an angiogram; it only showed 39% blockage of the same artery. The cardiologist thought that perhaps the blockage resulted from that neck surgery, in my early childhood, where the doctor had cut an artery as he removed the cyst; they were in the same part of the neck. **He also said that HRT can cause cardiovascular problems**. He told me to take and aspirin a day and to be checked periodically. I could not take the aspirin. He also restarted medicine for mitral valve prolapse; I had not taken that medicine for years. I took it for a short while, and stopped again because of the side effects.

<u>1998. November.</u> I went back to a gynecologist that I had seen much earlier, whom I had liked very much. I would have chosen him to do my hysterectomy had he been on my insurance plan at the time. He was now on the plan. I gave him my post-hysterectomy hormone history. I told him about the combination treatment of Tri-est/progesterone. I said that I had not had perfect results with them, either, but that I wanted to try natural hormones. He put me **back on Climara (a 7-day estradiol transdermal patch); that was "natural". Since the Sandra Cabot book had discussed estradiol patches, I was convinced to try it again.**

I had migraines before the end of the week, but the patch was better than the injections or the Premarin. (Nothing yet had helped the fibromyalgia pain as much as the Tri-est had.) I tried the patch for several months. During that time, I again started sporadically using the progesterone cream from the health food store. From my research, I learned that it may take up to three months to balance the hormones with the creams. The progest-erone cream helped the fatigue and body pain, but not the mi-graines. I was still unsure of its effects, and I had not told the gynecologist that I was using it.

1998, November. I kept the appointment with the endocrinologist. He agreed with the use of the Climara patch and added Premarin vaginal cream. I objected because of the bad side effects from the earlier use of the Premarin tablets; I did not use the cream.

1999, March 12. At another scheduled visit to the neurologist, I reported that I was still taking B12 shots, using hormone patches, and had stopped using the Elavil. I still had some migraines; the fibromyalgia was a little better; and the TMJ persisted and was worse in cold weather. My energy level was up, however.

1999, March 22. I told my gynecologist about the continued migraines and that I was experimenting with the progesterone cream. The Climara was not working well; he prescribed the Alora patch and testosterone cream (to be bought at a compounding pharmacy).

I did not know what a compounding pharmacy was. When I went to the pharmacy, I questioned them about Tri-est and progesterone; they assured me that they knew that various combinations of natural estrogens, progesterone, and sometimes testosterone had helped many women. **This made me realize that none of the hormones provided nearly as much relief from fibromyalgia pain as the Tri-Est and progesterone had given me in September. Besides, it occurred to me that I could not adjust the dosage of a patch like I could a cream.**

<u>1999, April.</u> I called the gynecologist. I told the nurse I wanted to try the Tri-est and progesterone cream again after talking with the compounding pharmacists. The doctor had no objection to phoning the prescription in for me. I started seeing results the first week. This saved my life. After about two months and some adjustments in dosages, I had no more hormonal migraines and my FMS symptoms had mostly disappeared. After several months on the program, I was able to stop using the testosterone because the libido and vaginal dryness problems were resolved.

<u>1999, July-August.</u> I had a long, depressing, and very traumatic ordeal as a result of the gallbladder surgery in February of 1998. Not long after surgery, I started having chronic diarrhea for which the internist prescribed Colestid. It stopped the diarrhea, but I was to find out after getting on the Tri-est and progesterone, over a year later, that the Colestid was causing some of the side effects that I attributed to FMS.

The bioidentical hormone program resolved the total-body-all-day pain of fibromyalgia, the migraines, the sleep problems, and the fibrofog. But I still had some leg pain and slight, nagging headaches off and on. These were not the horrible FMS symptoms, but they occurred daily, and they were distracting enough to warrant attention.

I noticed that when I skipped a day or two taking the Colestid, these leg pains and headaches did not occur, but I would have diarrhea on those days. This was a real dilemma. I reduced the two tablets of Colestid per day to just one; then I noticed that the leg pain and headaches occurred about an hour after taking the Colestid. I called the pharmacist; some of the **adverse reactions** of the medication include, among many others, musculoskeletal pain, aches and pains in the extremities, joint pains, femoral nerve pain. **It can also interfere with the absorption of fat-soluble vitamins. It binds with cholesterol, the main precursor of all hormones, so the hormones might be affected. Bingo!**

I went back to the doctor that did the gallbladder surgery because I wondered if something might have been wrong with the surgery—others I knew were not suffering as I was after the surgery. The surgeon prescribed Qustran Light and changed my long-standing prescription of Zantac to Prilosec. He ruled out other problems by ordering tests.

The side effects of the Questran Light were more severe and more numerous than the ones from the Colestid, and they included hormonal symptoms including hot flashes. I took the Questran Light for about four weeks hoping that some of the side effects would subside after a while. Meanwhile, I researched the side effects and drug interactions of Questran. **Questran can delay or reduce the absorption of certain medications, including estrogens and progestins.** It sometimes interferes with fat digestion and absorption and prevents absorption of the fat soluble vitamins A, D, E, and K, so taking these parenterally (other than by mouth) is suggested.

I went back to the internist because I thought he might know more about hormones than the surgeon. In light of my list, he agreed that my symptoms could possibly have been from the Colestid earlier, and now from the Questran; he prescribed Carafate. It did not prevent the diarrhea.

I was determined; there must be some way to stop this without so many side effects. I called the Dr. Mary Show (the WTIX radio show mentioned earlier) and asked for the best remedy for diarrhea after gallbladder surgery. His suggestion was paragoric, which my doctor got for me; it did not work either, so after a two-week trial, I gave that one up, too. The internal doctor and the surgeon agreed that I should see a gastroenterologist.

1999, July 12. In a scheduled visit to the neurologist, I was able to report that the fibromyalgia was better with the use of natural hormones. The knots in the legs were gone and I was not suffering from fatigue. He was encouraging and supportive when I told him I was writing this book. I had decreased medications: Xanax (.25) as needed, Lorcet as needed for pain, Questran, and Prilosec for the digestive problems caused by Questran.

1999, August 31-October. I was still looking for a medication to solve the chronic diarrhea resulting from gallbladder surgery. I saw the same gastroenterologist who had done the two latest colonoscopies. He prescribed Kutrase (an enzyme preparation). He ordered an endoscopy to check for Celiac Sprue disease; the test date was to be two weeks later on September 9. He said that if the Kutrase did not work, he would again suggest Questran Light. I brought up the side effects list; he seemed put off. He said that Questran should not cause any of the problems listed as side effects; those side effects are very rare; all medicines say that; he said that I should ignore the list. I then asked about the aspartame in the Questram Light; he appeared to think it was rediculous to raise the question.

On the way home, I stopped at an integrative medical clinic for their advice; they gave me a Meyers Cocktail, a shot of vitamins that lasts about a week. They also suggested I take acidophilus and natural enzymes. I decided to try the Kutrase first in order to get a good reading in the upcoming test; I did not take acidophilus or the natural enzymes just yet.

The Kutrase did not prevent diarrhea, and it caused stomach pain. After about a week, I became dehydrated. Also, I had severe heartburn, fever, stomach pains, and severe headache. Besides, the diarrhea was so bad that nothing I ate stayed with me for more than a few minutes. I went to the emergency room. They gave me intravenous fluids, Lomotil, and a Nubane shot (for headache). The emergency doctor suggested admittance to the hospital, but my insurance company refused, requiring instead that I be treated as an outpatient. I was home only a few hours when the diarrhea and stomach pains were back.

The gastroenterologist had already told me that Questran Light was his next choice if the Kutrase did not work so I took the Qustran Light that I already had at home. This time the Questran Light stopped only about half of the bouts of diarrhea. It also did not stop the stomachache, heartburn, blurred vision, weakness, headache, and in two days I was dehydrated again.

I called the gastroenterologist to report the situation. I told him my symptoms and asked if he might give me a vitamin shot, since I could not keep anything in my system and since the side effects for Questran Light mentioned vitamin depletion. He reluctantly agreed; he would call my local emergency room with instructions for the vitamin shot. I went in so dehydrated again that they barely could find veins for the vitamin and fluid treatments. The next day the headache and the weakness were better, and some of the other symptoms were beginning to subside, but I still had diarrhea significant enough to need attention, and I still had low fever.

At this point, I also worried that the upcoming test might show Celiac Sprue disease. I had two of the symptoms, rapid weight loss (25 pounds in three weeks) and diarrhea, so I called the nurse who agreed that I should avoid wheat products until the test. I then called a woman whose name was given me by the health food store and who had Celiac Sprue disease. She became my angel; she shared knowledge and went with me to the health food store to show me supplements to buy for the disease. (Her support was so meaningful to me; it made me realize the importance of my own sharing of knowledge with other fibromites.) I also got the natural enzymes and the acidophilus prescribed earlier by the integrative medical doctor.

That evening, about 6 P.M., I took the acidophilus in tea, and another dose of Questran Light. The Questran Light choked me, and I could not breathe for several seconds. By about 7:30 P.M., my throat and all the way down into my stomach began to burn severely. Rolaids did not help. I burned all night. At noon the next day, and again at supper, I took the scheduled doses of Questran because I feared being dehydrated from the diarrhea again. The burning increased in severity and began to include my tongue and the inside of my mouth. I was burning so badly that I could not sleep; I chewed ice all night, and paced the floor. I had other symptoms, too—blurred vision, weakness, low fever, and extreme depression.

I called the gastroenterologist the next morning. It was the weekend, so I talked to the doctor on call. I wanted to see him, but he told me just to take two Zantac at a time, instead of the prescribed one, until the endoscopy test date, a few days away. I was to continue the Questran Light.

The pain was unbearable, so I went in to see the gastroenterologist two days before the endoscopy. I was there as they opened, but they sent me to the emergency room instead. The doctor gave me an antacid cocktail. The nurse gave me some prescriptions for colon spasms and Axid for burning. The antacid cocktail gave me diarrhea as I had told the nurse it would. She said that was all they could do; I could wait to see the gastroenterologist that afternoon if I wished.

I did wait to see the gastroenterologist. He examined me, then he told me to go home and to continue the Questran Light and the Zantac until the endoscopy two days later. I was so sick; I could not believe that they would not admit me to the hospital. Nobody believed how sick I was. I truly thought that I would die before the two days until the endoscopy passed.

I did go home and I continued the medications. The burning continued all the while. I had followed the very bland diet suggested after the first episode of dehydration, so I was living on water, rice, jello, potatoes, and baked fish.

The endoscopy showed the doctor no obvious problems, but he intended to send the test to a lab, and the results would be back in a week. He told me that he thought that the burning was caused by anxiety. (A side effect of Questran is anxiety.) My husband asked what we should do; he told me to consult a psychiatrist and walked away.

1999, September 27. I became extremely depressed. My sister contacted a counselor. When I saw him, he suggested Zoloft in the morning and Trazodone at night. I took them; they aggravated the diarrhea again. He gave me a relaxation tape. He suggested a second opinion from another gastroenterologist.

A week later, I had an appointment with another gastroenterologist. He consulted by phone with my neurologist. His immediate reaction to my symptoms was to stop the Questran Light. He said that the burning is definitely a side effect, and that some people cannot tolerate the pain. He changed the Zoloft, which can cause diarrhea, to Prozac. He prescribed Elavil as an adjunct to the Prozac, and to slow down peristalsis. He told me to get back on the Colestid and to take just one Zantac twice a day. He spent a long time with me, and assured me of the likelihood of resolving this problem.

After just several days, the burning stopped. The depression abated in about two weeks. The Colestid prevented the diarrhea, and did not cause the usual leg pain and headaches until several weeks later, so for a short while I felt like a new person.

I decided that I would have to adjust to the Colestid and live with it because the doctors agree that bile is being dumped into the stomach, and that situation will not go away. I will always have some side effects from the Colestid. I will continue to look for a different way to solve this problem. For now, I have learned to take just one Colestid a day, and the diarrhea is under control most of the time. **I take it at least four to six hours away from the doses of hormone creams. I have improved more since I started taking a supplemental vitamin and mineral drink.**

1999, November 8. **On another scheduled visit to the neurologist, I could report that because of the bioidentical hormones I was back on track except for the effects of the Colestid. My depression was only minimal at this time. The migraines seemed to be controlled, so I did not need more Imitrex. I was exercising, getting back to work, and I was still writing the book.**

1999, November 12. I tripped and fell while walking to my car and caused severe pain in my lower back, neck, right shoulder, and arm. I already had bulging disks, and this fall caused me to worry that I may have ruptured one. I went to the chiropractor and also had myofascial release massage. These did not stop the neck, shoulder, or arm pain, but they helped the back pain somewhat.

2000, February-March. I had a MRI of my neck and back. It showed a herniated disk. It caused pain in the neck, right shoulder, and right arm. Options included surgery or an epidural. **The doctor favored the epidural in order to avoid surgery. I had the epidural injection that had cortisone in it. It caused an FMS flare-up with hormone imbalance symptoms, which I had not suffered for almost a year. I put my victory plan into full force, and the symptoms abated in about a month—that was very fast compared to earlier experiences.**

The epidural did not help the herniated disk; I am now considering surgery. I am looking for an alternative for this because I have learned from the past to try everything else before surgery.

The doctor is considering a laparoscopy to make sure that there are no problems from the gallbladder surgery before he allows neck surgery—I will have to be able to absorb supplements after surgery.

2000, April 6. I got a second opinion about the neck problem from a surgeon. He recommended surgery after viewing the MRI. He also prescribed a RS-4M Muscle Stimulator. It did not help the neck problem, but it did help pain in the lower back and the hip that resulted from the fall.

2000.April 20. I revisited my rheumatologist to tell him about my success with the fibromyalgia. I wanted to get his suggestions concerning the possible surgery for the herniated disk and its effects on my fibromyalgia. He prescribed the anti-inflammatory Vioxx for the disk problems and jaw pain. I could not take the medicine because of its side effects.

2000, May. I recently had to take antibiotics that caused me to have another few weeks of diarrhea—I failed to take the acidophilus. I had to get back on Elavil for two weeks, and Prozac. **Medicines I now take are Zantac 150; Lorcet, as needed; Xanax .25, twice daily; Prozac 20mg., once in the morning; and the Colestid. I also use the Progesterone and Tri-Est creams. Were it not for the gallbladder surgery problems, I would not need the Colestid or the Prozac. I will always have weather-related jaw pain because of the damage done to my jaw. Also, I have disk problems that will continue to affect me. Thanks to the bioidentical hormones, I no longer have the lifelong migraine headaches. I've learned to control my FMS pain and prevent flare-ups as long as I follow my victory plan.** I am very thankful that I searched and did not give up on having a normal life again.

2000, June. The latest development in my health is MSM, Methylsulfonyl-methane, an organic form of sulfur. The healing properties of MSM are just beginning to be fully identified. In New Orleans I met Susan Bernecker, the distributor of the Q-Knows brand of MSM. She suggested that I take the oral flavored MSM and use the massage cream as well. I have only used it for two weeks, and I do feel some improvement in my shoulder and arm pain caused by the herniated disk. It rained today, and the weather-related jaw pain that I usually have before any weather change did not bother me. That is a big change. Susan sent me a note in answer as to why this improvement has occurred. She said:

> MSM has demonstrated ability to alleviate pain associated with systemic inflammatory disorders. The nerves that sense pain are mainly located in the soft tissue of our bodies. Many types of pain can be attributed to pressure differential involving the cells that make up tissue. When outside pressure drops, cells swell and become inflamed. Nerves register the inflammation and we experience pain symptoms. Use of MSM (powdered for better absorption) has been shown to restore flexibility to the protein layer of cell walls, allowing fluids to pass through the tissue more easily. This softens the tissue and helps to equalize pressure thereby reducing, if not totally eliminating, the cause of the pain. By equalizing the cell pressure, MSM treats the cause of inflammation, unlike aspirin, which would treat the symptom by shutting off the nerve

For so many years I have taken so many anti-inflammatory drugs that my stomach rebels every time I take them now. Susan said that MSM is a good remedy for mucous membrane inflammation in the digestive tract. I have to say that the Colestid side effects seem milder since I started drinking the MSM in water.

For more information or to order the product, contact
Susan Bernecker at (504) 838-9881,
e-mail at susanbernecker@hotmail.com.
or visit her website at www.susanbernecker.com

Afterword

I spent many unproductive years searching for relief from the pain of fibromyalgia. Finally, I have found some answers that have given my life back to me. I will always have to consider this disease in making plans. But, now I can at least make plans and enjoy carrying them out with little or no pain. I can now set longer and more interesting goals, like writing a book, that include activities other than pain management and getting through the day. I could not do that before. As I said, I have reduced the pain of fibromyalgia by eighty to ninety percent. Now I control FMS; it does not control me anymore.

I have had some setbacks. All the years of assault on my body from the fibromyalgia and from the countless treatments have made me super sensitive to almost everything that happens in my body. The bouts with Questran, Colestid, and cortisone injections have delayed the completion of our hard work. This just shows how completely negative events can disrupt the life of a fibromite even when the FMS has been brought under control. However, it took much less time to recuperate from these compared to similar events earlier in my life. I feel that I have demonstrated how effective a good victory plan can be. The experience proves to me, beyond a shadow of a doubt, that my FMS is caused from an imbalance of hormones and that only the bioidentical hormones are beneficial in correcting the imbalance and controlling the FMS.

Several points should be emphasized because of their importance for anyone on the fibromyalgia trip. First, don't give up; keep looking; be persistent. Be the captain of your own team. Take responsibility for your condition; read about it and study it. Keep in touch with other fibromites. If something works for you, then use it no matter what others may think. Remember that others have succeeded in controlling FMS and that means you can, too.

Learn to manage stress by anticipating and preventing it. Learn the techniques that help you to relax. Find methods to alleviate fear of situations that you cannot control. Practice and visualize yourself in control.

Listen to signals from your body. Learn your triggers and bodily responses to various stimuli. Start to take note of times and types of internal changes or messages. Many times pain can be stopped or avoided if you recognize the onset early and take the necessary actions. Try relaxation exercises, meditation, massage, magnet therapy, or others mentioned here. You may find more on your own.

Keep a diary (see back of book). Write down your reactions to everything—medications, stress responses, exercises. This done on a daily basis helped me to see and to analyze patterns; it helped me to formulate my victory plan.

I could have avoided many bad experiences if I had asked more questions in the beginning instead of simply relying on the information offered to me. Check out all medications, treatments, or surgeries very thoroughly before you submit to them. Unnecessary treatments, or incorrect ones, are wasteful of time and money. As I learned, they can also be hurtful and harmful. Use the least medication or least invasive treatment possible to effect cure or improvement. Some doctors prefer one treatment to another simply because they are more familiar with it and it has worked for them before, but that does not necessarily mean that it is the best treatment for your condition at the time. Ask the doctor; ask the pharmacist about every medication and its possible side effects. Read the information paper given when the prescription is filled. What will this treatment or medication do? What are the side effects? Will it react with or interfere with other medications being used? What percentage of patients finds relief using this treatment? What percentage of patients suffers bad side effects? What would happen if nothing at all were done (it has become law in New Jersey for doctors to give this information to patients). What natural, alternative, or other treatments could be considered? Ask the pharmacist for the manufacturer information on each drug; this is more complete than the summary given out with the prescription, and it can be very helpful.

Be willing to consider alternative treatments instead of or along with conventional ones, but get professional help in using them. This is not always easy. In some areas, few doctors are trained to use alternative treatments, and many doctors do not even accept them as valid; they are unwilling to use such treatments. This is improving, though; there are even doctors in New Orleans who offer magnet therapy now. More doctors are beginning to use both conventional and alternative therapies; thus we now more often hear the new terms integrative or complementary medicine—and we did not hear them at all just a few years ago.

Realize that a treatment that seems not to work may simply need adjustment. Work with the doctor and try different amounts and timing of doses. Try medications with food and then without food unless stated otherwise in the directions. This all takes time and patience, but it can lead to a successful treatment.

Choose your doctor carefully; pay attention to your intuition. Check credentials and track records. Ask friends. Find out his attitude and success rate for treating fibromyalgia. If the doctor appears demeaning or uncommunicative, find the exit. You may have to search and search and search until you find a doctor who will work with you and value you as an intelligent, capable human being. If you have to travel out of your area to find such a doctor, you can deduct many of the expenses from your taxes. When you do find the one, you make sure to work very closely with him or her.

Just remember that winning the battle of overcoming FMS doesn't come overnight. It takes a lot of love, understanding, and patience from you and from your family. Remember that you have to crawl before you walk, and you have to walk before you run. I sincerely hope this helps each and every one of you have an easier journey in conquering and coping with FMS and its flare-ups.

My web site address is **www.iconqueredfibromyalgia.com.** Please visit me there and offer feedback, or you can e-mail me at fmspam@aol.com. I would love to get news of your experiences using the methods suggested here.

NEWS FLASH! News from the Internet. My brother-in-law directed me to health.excite.com (WebM.D., Inc.) medical news. L.A. McKeown tells about new research on fibromyalgia. The article says a lot, but the bottom line is that researchers think that fibromyalgia may be caused by too high or too low hormone levels due to the fact that the HPA axis is damaged. Besides the HPA axis, the researchers suggest that damage in the autonomic nervous system may be a factor. These studies are from Harvard and Brigham and Women's Hospital; some have been published in the *American Journal of Medicine.* And a Tulane/Ochsners fibromyalgia study is underway at this time. The "big guns" are interested in our plight. This is very encouraging news.

Books and Resources

The more I educated myself, the more I was able to establish meaningful doctor-patient relationships, and the better able I was to cope and to conquer. I then knew, and was able to ask, the questions that got valuable information. I gained insights into new possibilities for my situation.

Studying may seem hard to do, especially for a person who already feels miserable. When you have FMS, the task of staying comfortable seems to take almost all of your stamina, focus, and time. Therefore, the need to study can seem like a daunting task that you just do not think you have the energy, the time, or the resources to do. Furthermore, there is the fear that you may find out horrible things. There may be fear that the remedies you do find will cost hundreds of dollars and/or hours. If you are depressed, you may feel that nothing has worked, so why go looking for more "pie in the sky"? In my age group there is that cultural habit that tells us never to question the doctor; he is the expert; just leave everything to the doctor; no need to study, it just gets in the way. And, of course, there is often that old human tendency to stick your head in the sand. Study anyway! From experience I can tell you that just one piece of encouraging new information can give you unbelievable courage and lift.

My experience studying FMS has taught me some things about my ability to cope with large quantities of new information. Some of the books are so detailed and technical that they are frightening at first. At times, reading some of these long, technical books overwhelmed and depressed me. I found it better to start with shorter and more generalized articles and books. Going from very general, like the Parade article, to more and more sophisticated works, like the Starlanyl book, worked best for me. If the book seems too hard or too depressing in any way, put it down and get one that is either shorter or less complex--you don't need more confusion in your life. Do not discard the "hard" book because you will most certainly want to use it later on. Also, do not give yourself overwhelming assignments—you don't have to read every line in every book. The best books have great indices, so you can look up a specific topic and read just two or three pages on that subject.

Several books and other resources have been mentioned and quoted in this book. I encourage you to read all of them and to find others that pertain to FMS. As more doctors and sufferers recognize FMS, there will be more and more helpful literature to be found. Keep on reading.

The following resources helped me a lot:

Cabot, Sandra, M.D. 1995. *Smart Medicine for Menopause.* Garden City Park, NY: Avery Publishing Group.

This was one of the first books I read after my hysterectomy. If I had read this book before the surgery, I never would have agreed to a total hysterectomy. This book opened my eyes to the fact that hormones must be balanced on an individual basis and that HRT can have dramatic effects on the body.

Crook, William G., M.D. 1995. *Chronic Fatigue Syndrome and the Yeast Connection.* Jackson, TN: Professional Books.

I still follow his suggestions for using acidophilus to maintain "healthy" bacteria in the digestive system.

Grout, Pam. 1996. *Jumpstart Your Metabolism.* New York: Fireside.

Grout's suggestions are presented in a very interesting way, and they seem to work very well. I've used quite a few of them. I refer to this book often; it is excellent to help you relax (and lose weight).

International Journal of Pharmaceutical Compounding (Vol. 2, No. 1, Jan./Feb. 1998), Interview on HRT: Christiane Northrup, M.D., FACOG., (12-17).

The article mentions her newsletter and books. I have not yet read them, but she seems to be so "cutting edge" that I want to see what she has to say.

Lee, John R., M.D., Jesse Hanley, M.D., and Viginia Hopkins. 1999. *What Your Doctor May* Not *Tell You About Pre-menopause.* New York: Warner Books, Inc.

______and Virginia Hopkins. 1996. *What Your Doctor May* Not *Tell You About Menopause.* New York: Warner Books, Inc.

Every woman should have a copy of one of these books. They explain so many conditions that women—and men—suffer. The explanations are very easy to understand. They tell just how to use the progesterone cream. If you read these books, you will want to recommend them to friends. I believe the information here explains the root of my FMS. In fact, the books explain many of the illnesses that affect our whole society; they are based on good scientific studies by reputable researchers. There are lists of addresses and contacts for organizations and businesses.

Merck Manual. 1999. Editors, Mark H. Beers, M.D. and Robert Berkow, M.D., 17th ed. Rahway, N.J.: Merck & Co., Inc.

Reader's Digest Family Guide to Natural Medicine. 1993. Ed. Alma E. Guinness. The Reader's Digest Association. (99).

Rosenfeld, Isadore, M.D. 1999. When you just hurt all over. *Parade. 18 July, 16.*

This article was very comforting because it was the first time I had seen such affirmation in the popular press by a medical doctor. That felt like real progress to me.

Starlanyl, Devin J., M.D. and Mary Ellen Copeland, M.S., M.A. 1996. *Fibromyalgia & Chronic Myofascial Pain Syndrome, A Survival Manual.* Oakland, CA: New Harbinger Publications, Inc. 9th reprint, 1999. New Harbinger Publications, Inc.

My neurologist suggested this book; it is an excellent guide, the most complete I've found. It is one that I suggest for use as a reference to look up special topics until you are ready for an in depth study. This book would be helpful if you were to read nothing but the preface and the bibliography. Starlanyl has FMS herself, and so does Copeland, so as they write, they put many myths firmly and humorously in their places. It is a superior tool to take to the doctor because it is presented in scientific form and has an extensive reference list taken largely from medical literature. It has numerous illustrations. Tender points versus trigger points—their book includes excellent and detailed illustrations and descriptions on the characteristics of tender points, and a whole chapter on trigger points. The book offers a newsletter and a video to help sustain and teach methods for controlling pain.

Taber, Clarence Wilbur. 1965. *Taber's Cyclopedic Medical Dictionary.* 10th ed. Philadelphia, PA: F. A. Davis Company.

Taber's Cyclopedic Medical Dicionary. 1997 ed. Clayton L. Thomas, M.D, M.P.H. 18th ed. Philadelphia, PA: F. A. Davis Company.

Vliet, Elizabeth Lee, M.D. 1995. *Screaming to be Heard, Hormonal Connections that Women Suspect...and Doctors Ignore.* New York: M. Evans and Company, Inc.

Another book suggested to me by the neurologist. This is a very complete book for women's health. It agrees with my theory on hormonal connections to various health problems. This book can help women put their bodies back on the right track for healthier lives.

Williamson, Miryam Ehrlich. 1996. *fibromyalgia: a comprehensive approach: what you can do about chronic pain and fatigue*. With a foreword by David A. Nye, M.D. New York: Walker and Company.

Easy to read, this a good reference for your early studies. Included are very good suggestions for nutrition, supplementation, and detoxification. A complete list of associated conditions is included. Also, there is a section on what you should tell friends, co-workers, and bosses about your condition.

Your Guide to Living Well with Fibromyalgia. 1997. The Arthritis Foundation. Atlanta, Ga: Longstreet Press, Inc.

My Diary:

Many Doctors will find this Diary to be helpful in evaluating your condition. I also found it to be helpful in dealing with my fibromyalgia on a daily basis. I have not only included questions to ask yourself, but also some advice to help you along the way. This way of keeping a diary helped me to look at my situation on paper and realize that I still had a lot to be thankful for and that there were many others with diseases much worse than mine. I always took time to pray to God and ask Him for his help and guidance and thank Him for any progress I made along the way.

Here is a Seven Day Diary to help you get started:

- What time did I wake up? How did I sleep?

Day one:

Day two:

Day three:

Day four:

Day five:

Day Six:

Say Seven:

- How did I feel? (Any fatigue, stiffness, headaches, muscle pains, hot flashes, irritable bowel, etc...)
  (Was I happy, depressed, anxious, etc...)

<u>Day one:</u>

<u>Day two:</u>

<u>Day three:</u>

<u>Day four:</u>

<u>Day five:</u>

Day Six:

Day Seven:

- What was the first thing I did today?

Day one:

Day two:

Day three:

Day four:

Day five:

Day Six:

<u>Day Seven:</u>

- What did I eat and drink for breakfast? Did I feel any different after eating? Record stomach pains or unusual digestive problems from any foods. You may be allergic to some foods, such as diary products, caffeine, orange juice, etc... Some foods give patients headaches, muscle pains, irritable bowel, or more arthritic type pains.

Day One:

Day two:

Day three:

Day four:

Day five:

Day Six:

Day Seven:

- Did I take any morning medicines? What time? Record any change in symptoms especially within the next hour or two. Check side effects of medications with the pharmacist; don't just rely on the paper given to you from the pharmacy because it only lists a few of the side effects. Should your medications be taken with or without food?

Day one:

Day two:

Day three:

Day four:

Day five:

Day Six:

Day Seven:

- Did I take any morning vitamins or herbs? What time? Record any change in symptoms especially within the next hour or two. Make sure not to take medications, herbs, and vitamins all together. This can sometimes cause some dangerous side effects. Some vitamins and herbs can block absorption of many medications. Some medications can block absorption of certain vitamins. Some herbs and medications should never be taken together as they can cause death.

Day one:

Day two:

Day three:

Day four:

Day five:

Day Six:

Day Seven:

- Did I do any stretches? Note what kind, how many and for how long. Was I comfortable while stretching?
  How did I feel? Was I sore before or after?

<u>Day one:</u>

<u>Day two:</u>

<u>Day three:</u>

<u>Day four:</u>

<u>Day five:</u>

Day Six:

Day Seven:

- Did I walk on the treadmill or do any bicycle exercising? How did I feel? How long did I exercise? Was I short of breath? Was I getting my heart rate up?

<u>Day one:</u>

<u>Day two:</u>

<u>Day three:</u>

<u>Day four:</u>

<u>Day five:</u>

Day Six:

Day Seven:

- Did I walk around the block outside. Some people prefer to walk outdoors and I found this to be beneficial especially for depression. Take time to look around at God's creations. Record some happy and refreshing comments about your walk.

Day one:

Day two:

Day three:

Day four:

Day five:

Day Six:

Day Seven:

- Midmorning—How did I feel? Any snacks, or medications? Any pain?

Day one:

Day two:

Day three:

Day four:

Day five:

Day Six:

Day Seven:

- What did I eat and drink for lunch? Did I take any medications, vitamins, or herbs? How did I feel? Have I had any stressful events take place so far today?

Day one:

Day two:

Day three:

Day four:

Day five:

Day Six:

Day Seven:

- How did I feel this afternoon? Was I doing any exercises or stretches while going through the day? Try to relax the mind and the body through meditation and relaxation techniques. What have I done to relax myself? Follow examples in the book.

Day one:

Day two:

Day three:

Day four:

Day five:

Day Six:

Day Seven:

- What have I had to eat and drink for dinner? Have I taken any medications, vitamins, or herbs? How did I feel? Any pain, fatigue, headaches, etc...

Day one:

Day two:

Day three:

Day four:

Day five:

Day Six:

Day Seven:

- Have I done any more exercises or stretches? Remember do not exercise two hours before bedtime as this may disturb your sleep.

Day one:

Day two:

Day three:

Day four:

Day five:

Day Six:

Day Seven:

- Bedtime——What have I done for myself today? Is there at least one thing that I have accomplished and I am proud of?

<u>Day one:</u>

<u>Day two:</u>

<u>Day three:</u>

<u>Day four:</u>

<u>Day five:</u>

Day Six:

Day Seven:

- Am I tired and do I feel like I can go to sleep? Have I taken any medications, vitamins, or herbs. It is best to take most vitamins in the daytime as they may disturb your sleep. Do I have any pain, anxiety, or depression?

Day one:

Day two:

Day three:

Day four:

Day five:

Day Six:

Day Seven:

- Is my bed comfortable? Am I sleeping on the right kind of pillow? Sleeping on your stomach is the worst position a person can go to sleep in. Do I need any sleep aids such as an icepack, mattress pad, magnets, etc...?

Day one:

Day two:

Day three:

Day four:

Day five:

Day Six:

Day Seven:

Notes

Notes

Questions for my doctors!

Questions for my doctors!

We wish you all the best in health and happiness and may God's blessing be with each of you. Take some time to write a few encouraging comments about your progress
that you can share with others: